Preface

Color Guide to Neonatology is for use as an aid to clinical diagnosis for nurses, midwives, and undergraduate and postgraduate medical staff. It is not intended to be a comprehensive textbook of neonatal medicine and surgery but merely gives a brief outline of neonatal care and conditions that can be represented in clinical photographs.

We acknowledge the help of Mrs. Rosamund Brodie of the RPMS Institute of Obstetrics and Gynaecology, Queen Charlotte's and Chelsea Hospital, London, who took some of the photographs.

Contents

Mongolian blue spot

Incidence

Almost universal in non-white neonates. The condition is particularly obvious in Asian infants and occasionally occurs in white infants with dark hair.

Clinical features

Slate gray or bluish pigmentation, usually in the lumbosacral region (Figs. 1 and 2), but may occur anywhere on the trunk or limbs (Fig. 3).

Significance

None, except may be mistaken for bruising by the inexperienced.

Course and prognosis

Gradually becomes less obvious as the infant grows older.

Erythema toxicum

Synonyms

Toxic erythema, urticaria of the newborn, eosinophil rash.

Incidence

Extremely common. Most newborn infants are affected in the first week of life. It is not seen in preterm infants.

Etiology

Unknown.

Pathology

Vesicles are full of eosinophils.

Clinical features

Widespread, fluctuating erythematous maculopapular rash (Fig. 4), usually beginning after birth at any time in the first week. Individual lesions consist of a white central papule surrounded by an erythematous flare.

Significance

None, except may occasionally be mistaken for infectious pustules.

Course

Disappears spontaneously.

Management

None required.

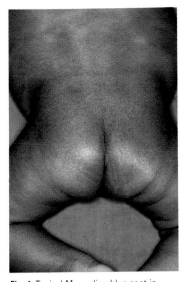

Fig. 1 Typical Mongolian blue spot in lumbosacral region.

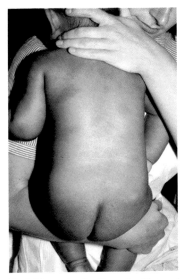

Fig. 2 More extensive Mongolian blue spot.

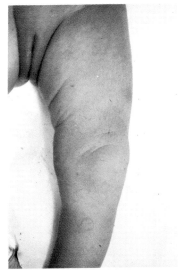

Fig. 3 Mongolian blue spot around the knee.

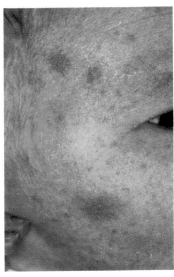

Fig. 4 Erythema toxicum on the face.

Vernix caseosum

Incidence

Common.

Clinical features

Slimy, ointment-like white substance on the skin of some infants at birth. It is usually found around the face (Fig. 5) and ears and in the folds of the neck or groin (Fig. 6) but is occasionally liberally caked all over the body. <u>Vernix is sometimes stained by meconium if there was fetal distress sometime before birth.</u> Vs Erythema toxicum Not in Pic

Significance

None. Vernix is more common toward the end of gestation but tends to disappear after term.

Course

Dries and flakes off within a few hours after birth.

Management

None required.

Vascular phenomena

Incidence

Very common.

Etiology

Innocent manifestation of vasomotor instability or immaturity.

Clinical features

1. <u>Peripheral cyanosis</u> is very common in the first 48 h after birth. It occurs in the extremities and around the mouth. There is no central cyanosis.
2. <u>Harlequin color change</u> is a very rare but dramatic color change with vivid midline demarcation of color (Fig. 7). The infant is red on one side of the trunk and pale on the other side.

Management

None required.

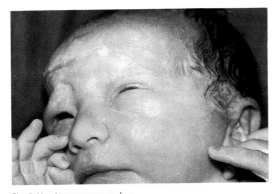

Fig. 5 Vernix caseosum on face.

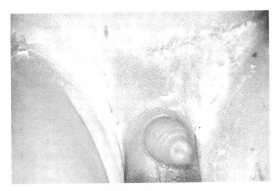

Fig. 6 Vernix caseosum in the groin.

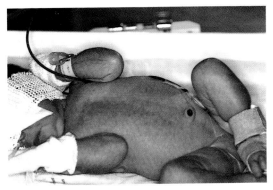

Fig. 7 Harlequin vascular phenomenon.

Milia and Epstein pearls

Synonym	Milk spots.
Incidence	Very common; seen in 40–50% of newborn infants.
Pathology	Milia are hypertrophic sebaceous glands. Epstein pearls are epidermal cysts.
Clinical features	Milia are fine white spots seen on the nose (Fig. 8) and cheeks. Epstein pearls occur as a cluster of several white spots in the mouth at the junction of the soft and hard palate in the midline (Fig. 9). Less commonly, they occur on the alveolar margin or on the prepuce.
Significance	None, but occasionally mistaken for infection.
Course and prognosis	Disappear spontaneously.

Ranula

Incidence	Uncommon.
Clinical features	Superficial mucous retention cyst in the anterior part of the floor of the mouth, under the tongue (Fig. 10). Deeper cysts may occur in relation to the submandibular or sublingual ducts.
Management	Often disappear spontaneously. Large cysts may occasionally interfere with feeding, and surgery may then be indicated (marsupialization).

Natal teeth

Incidence	Uncommon, but there is often a family history of similar teeth.
Clinical features	Commonly occur in the central lower incisor region (Fig. 11) and are usually only loosely attached.
Management	Best removed early to prevent aspiration or ulceration of the tongue. Extraction will not deplete the permanent dentition.

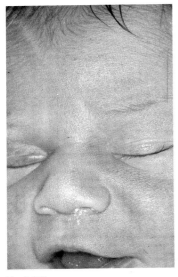

Fig. 8 Milia on nose.

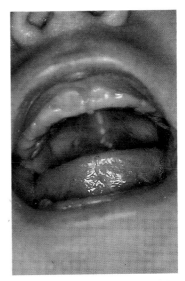

Fig. 9 Epstein pearls in the midline of the palate.

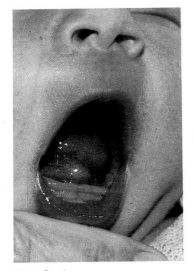

Fig. 10 Ranula.

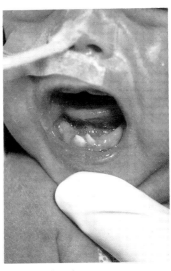

Fig. 11 Natal teeth.

Simple nevus

Synonym	Stork bite nevus.
Incidence	Very common; seen in 30–50% of infants.
Pathology	Capillary hemangioma.
Clinical features	Bright pink macular capillary hemangioma seen on the eyelids, bridge of the nose, upper lip (Fig. 12), and nape of the neck (Fig. 13). On the forehead, there is sometimes a V-shaped lesion said in folklore to be the mark of the stork's beak. Simple nevi do not blanch on pressure.
Significance	None.
Course and prognosis	All simple nevi on the face disappear spontaneously in the first year. Those on the nape of the neck are usually permanent but never require treatment.

Sucking pad

Synonym	Sucking callus.
Incidence	Common.
Clinical features	Dry thickened epithelium of the mucous membranes of the lips (Fig. 14) in the first few weeks of life. They often form a discrete pad or callus.
Etiology	Unknown, but not related to pressure or trauma as they can occur in the absence of sucking and are often present at birth.
Significance	None.
Management	None required. They disappear spontaneously.

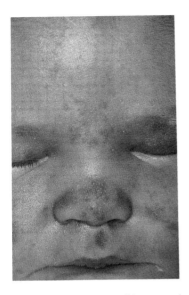

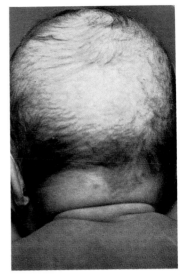

Fig. 12 Simple nevus on eyelids, nose, and upper lip.

Fig. 13 Simple nevus on nape of the neck.

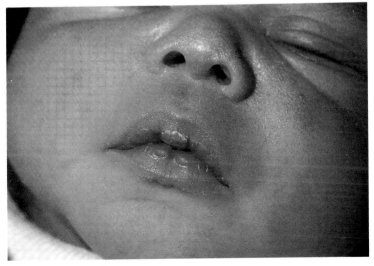

Fig. 14 Sucking pad on lip.

Hormonal manifestations: gynecomastia and vaginal bleeding

Incidence

Very common. Most newborn infants have palpable breast nodules, and 30–40% have obvious gynecomastia. Both sexes may have gynecomastia.

Etiology

Probably due to placental transfer of maternal estrogen, progesterone, and prolactin.

Clinical features

Breast enlargement, often with lactation (witch's milk), is present during the first weeks of life. In hormonal gynecomastia, there is no evidence of inflammation (Fig. 15). Erythema only occurs when the breast has become infected (mastitis). Vaginal bleeding, or a discharge of mucus (Fig. 16), occurs in some infants a few days after birth.

Course

Gradual involution of the breast tissue occurs but may take some months to disappear.

Management

No treatment is required for hormonal gynecomastia and vaginal bleeding. Reassurance and explanation of the physiologic nature of these events should be given to the parents. Do not squeeze the breasts to express milk. Antibiotics are only necessary if the breast becomes infected.

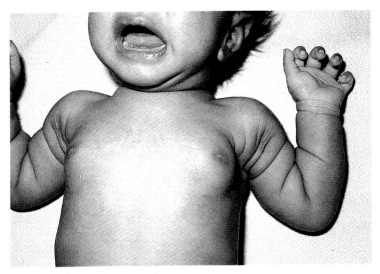

Fig. 15 Normal neonatal gynecomastia.

Duodenal oestrogen / precedated prola
procedole bbreost feedy

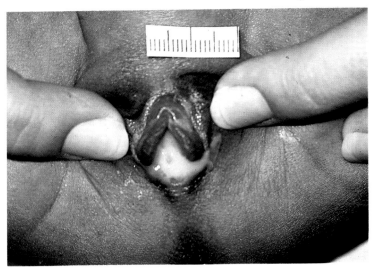

Fig. 16 Normal mucoid vaginal discharge.

Sacral pits and dimples

Incidence Common.

Clinical features Pits or dimples are often present over the sacrum (Fig. 17), and a prominent coccyx can often be palpated in the base.

Significance They are usually trivial and blind-ending. Fistulas can usually be excluded by careful inspection; otherwise, radiologic investigation may be necessary.

Associations Other midline abnormalities such as hemangioma, hairy nevi or lipomas may occur. They are usually situated higher on the back and may be associated with tethering of the cauda equina (diastatomyelia).

Management None required if fistula has been excluded.

Vulval tag

Incidence Common.

Clinical features A tag of mucous membrane is often present in the posterior vulval region of newborn female infants (Fig. 18). It is often long and pedunculated.

Significance None.

Course and prognosis Shrivels up and disappears spontaneously within a few days of birth.

Management None required.

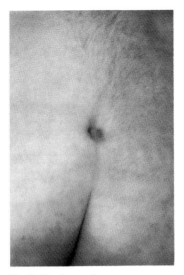

Fig. 17 Dimple over the sacrum.

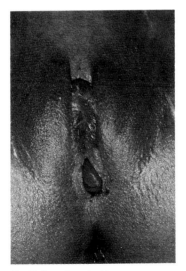

Fig. 18 Posterior vulval tag.

Umbilical cord

Clinical features

The umbilical cord usually has a fleshy translucent appearance in the first days after birth. It is sometimes stained yellow or greenish yellow with bilirubin in rhesus hemolytic disease or with meconium if there has been fetal distress. The normal umbilical cord contains two arteries and one vein (Fig. 19). A single umbilical artery may be associated with other congenital abnormalities.

Course

The cord gradually separates within 7–10 days after birth, either by dry gangrene (Fig. 20) or with a residual moist base (Fig. 21). Frank discharge or cellulitis with a red flare around the umbilicus indicates infection and requires treatment with systemic antibiotics after culture. Persistent serosanguineous discharge or a fleshy protuberance from the base may indicate the development of an umbilical granuloma. The presence of a vitello-intestinal remnant or persistent urachus should be excluded. A granuloma can be readily treated with the local application of silver nitrate or rarely by surgical excision.

Management

Gentle cleaning with a spirit swab is all that is required for the normal moist umbilical cord until spontaneous separation occurs. The application of topical antibiotics may actually delay separation. Prolonged adherence of the umbilical cord beyond 3 weeks of age has been associated with a rare disorder of granulocyte function.

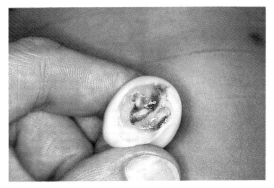

Fig. 19 Cut surface of umbilical cord showing two arteries and one vein.

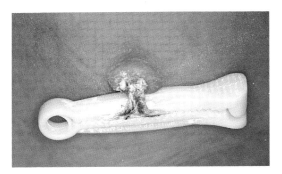

Fig. 20 Dry cord.

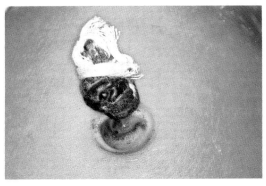

Fig. 21 Separating cord with a moist base.

Stools

Meconium

Sticky, tarry, greenish black stool (Fig. 22) passed by the newborn infant within the first 48 h after birth. Failure to pass meconium within 48 h of birth may indicate intestinal obstruction. Meconium is odorless and consists of mucus, epithelial debris, and bile from the gastrointestinal tract before feeding. Meconium may be passed by the fetus before birth if there is fetal distress. Inhalation of meconium results in pneumonitis with severe respiratory distress, and vigorous suction and resuscitation are indicated immediately after delivery before the first spontaneous breath.

Changing stool

With the onset of feeding, the stools gradually change in color and consistency (Fig. 23). They become softer, greenish, and mixed with mucus for a few days.

Breast-fed baby's stools

Mustard yellow or greenish yellow and only a faint sweet odor. Breast-fed baby's stools are usually soft and semiformed (Fig. 24) but are sometimes liquid. Frequency varies, but they are often passed after or during each feed.

Bottle-fed baby's stools

Usually firmer and browner and passed less frequently than those of a breast-fed infant. The appearance and odor vary considerably, but in general they are more like a normal adult stool.

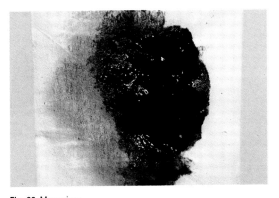

Fig. 22 Meconium.

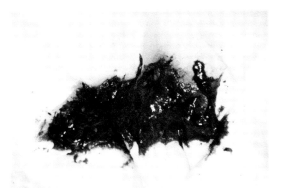

Fig. 23 Changing stool.

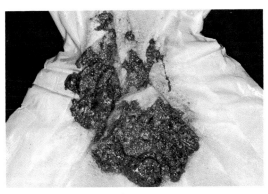

Fig. 24 Breast-fed baby's stool.

Jaundice

Very common. About 50% of full-term infants and 80% of preterm babies are visibly jaundiced by 3–5 days of age.

- *Early jaundice* occurring within 24–48 h of birth is usually due to abnormal hemolysis, infection, or bruising from birth trauma and is usually pathologic (cord or initial screen bilirubin ≥ 5 mg/dl, or a level of >10 mg/dl at 12 h of age, or any type of conjugated hyperbilirubinemia).
- *Physiologic jaundice* appears after 48 h of birth and usually settles within 7–10 days.
- *Prolonged jaundice* lasting beyond 14 days is sometimes seen in normal preterm or breast-fed infants, but other conditions should be excluded, especially hypothyroidism, galactosemia, liver disease, red cell enzyme defects and biliary atresia.

Clinical features

Yellow staining of the skin (Fig. 25) and conjunctiva. Hepatosplenomegaly indicates the presence of abnormal hemolysis, infection, or a metabolic disorder and is not found in physiologic jaundice.

Significance

Very severe unconjugated hyperbilirubinemia may cause permanent brain damage (kernicterus) with athetoid cerebral palsy and sensorineural deafness.

Management

Investigation may be required if jaundice appears earlier than 48 h, is prolonged beyond 14 days, or is unusually high at any stage. Phototherapy (Fig. 26) or exchange transfusion may be required in some infants with high levels of plasma bilirubin. Exchange transfusion is reserved for those with rapidly rising bilirubin levels from hemolytic processes or overproduction or those at risk for kernicterus. Exchange levels are lower in critically ill or premature infants. Some jaundiced babies develop a curious bronze color under phototherapy (Fig. 27). This bronze coloring is particularly a risk with conjugated hyperbilirubinemia. If an infant requires phototherapy the following baseline laboratory studies should be obtained: mother's blood type and antibody screen, baby's blood type with screen (preferably, a direct antibody test or Coomb's test), hematocrit and reticulocyte count.

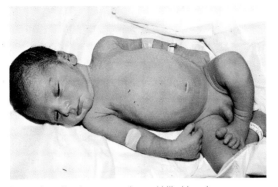

Fig. 25 Jaundice due to unconjugated bilirubinemia.

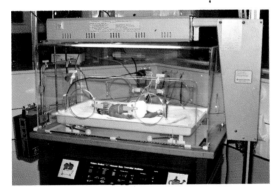

Fig. 26 Phototherapy.

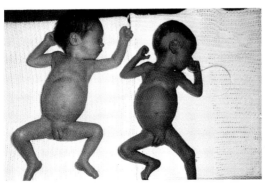

Fig. 27 Bronze baby syndrome with a normal baby.

Neonatal reflexes (1)

Occurrence

The normal newborn infant has a large number of primitive neurologic reflexes that disappear spontaneously during early infancy. The presence or absence may be useful in the assessment of gestational age and neurologic function. Delayed disappearance of certain primitive reflexes may be an early sign of cerebral palsy.

Moro or startle reflex

Clinical features

The infant is held supine, with trunk and head being supported from below. When the head and shoulders are suddenly allowed to fall back, a startle response with rapid abduction and extension of the upper limbs followed by slower abduction and flexion is elicited. The Moro reflex is often accompanied by a cry and may be demonstrated unintentionally when briskly placing an infant in the supine position (Fig. 28). Babies do not seem to like the reflex, so it should not be elicited as a routine procedure. The most common cause of an asymmetric Moro response is a fracture of the humerus or clavicle or a brachial plexus palsy.

Grasp reflexes

Flexion of the digits is a positive response to a finger being placed on the palmar surface of the base of the fingers (Fig. 29) or the plantar surface of the toes.

Sucking and rooting reflexes

Stroking the face around the mouth or cheek causes a reflex sucking (Fig. 30) and searching response. ➡

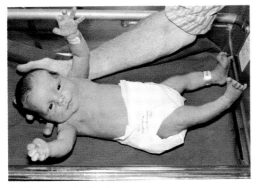

Fig. 28 Moro or startle reflex.

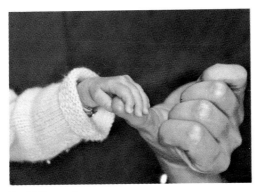

Fig. 29 Grasp reflex.

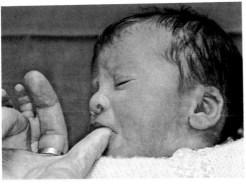

Fig. 30 Sucking response.

Neonatal reflexes (2)

Clinical features
(cont.)

Glabellar tap
A blink of the eyelids is produced in response to tapping the base of the nose.

Traction reflex
Pulling the infant up from the supine position by the wrists results in flexion of the arms and neck.

Placing reflex
If the foot is brought up gently under the edge of a surface, the leg is flexed and the baby places the foot on the surface.

Stepping reflex
When the sole of the foot is brought into contact with a surface, there is an automatic stepping movement (Fig. 31).

Galant reflex
If the posterior loin is stroked, the baby swings the buttock toward that side.

Asymmetric tonic neck reflex
If the head is turned laterally, there is extension of the arm and leg on the same side and flexion of the opposite arm and leg (Fig. 32).

Significance

Only very general conclusions can be drawn from examination of an infant for primitive reflexes. None of the reflexes is associated with a particular anatomic or pathologic lesion. Their presence or absence must be considered in association with the history, gestational age, and other aspects of the neurologic examination. Most primitive reflexes are extinguished by 4 months of age.

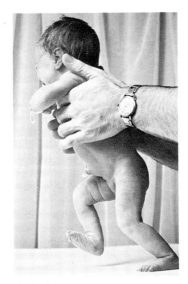

Fig. 31 Automatic stepping.

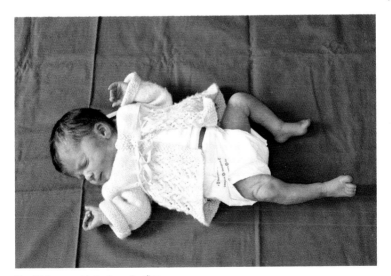

Fig. 32 Asymmetric tonic neck reflex.

Care of the full-term infant

Birth

If the baby is in good condition, it can be given immediately to the parents for them to hold and inspect. Some babies do not breathe by 2 min and need ventilation by intubation or bag and mask. Any meconium must be aspirated carefully from the respiratory tract.

Warmth

Hypothermia can easily occur and may cause further complications. The baby must be dried carefully and then wrapped and kept in a warm environment (Fig. 33). The infant's temperature should be measured on admission to the postnatal ward.

Feeding

There is a definite advantage in breast-feeding (Fig. 34), and this should begin in the delivery room. Supplements of infant formula should be strongly discouraged, especially if there is a family history of allergy.

Infection

Newborn babies are easily colonized with pathogenic organisms. All staff must pay particular attention to handwashing between touching babies. The umbilical cord is a favorite site for colonization; it should be left uncovered and treated with alcohol only.

Family relationships

The baby should not be taken away from the mother unless absolutely necessary and should be nursed next to the mother's bed. Everyone who works on a maternity floor should do their best to discourage any practice that interferes with the normal relationship of a mother and her baby.

Examination

A full medical examination of the infant should be performed within 24 h of birth to exclude major congenital abnormalities and to reassure the parents that the baby is well.

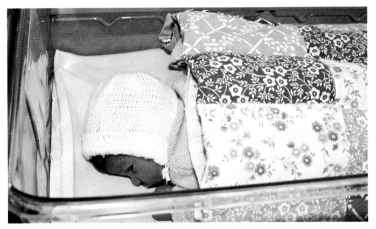

Fig. 33 The baby should be kept well wrapped and in a warm environment to prevent hypothermia.

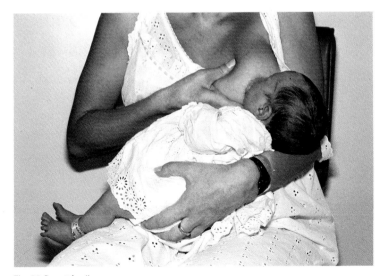

Fig. 34 Breast-feeding.

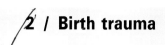

2 / Birth trauma

Molding of the head

Clinical features

Elongation and narrowing of the skull (Fig. 35) with overlapping of cranial sutures occurs as part of the normal birth process in most vaginal deliveries.

Course and prognosis

Normal shape of the head returns within a few days of birth.

Caput succedaneum

Clinical features

Subcutaneous edema and bruising of the presenting part (Fig. 36), usually the parietal or occipital region of the head. A caput is a diffuse, generalized soft tissue swelling that freely crosses suture lines.

Course and prognosis

The swelling is maximal immediately after birth and disappears spontaneously within a few days.

Cephalhematoma

Incidence

Less common than caput but still common.

Clinical features

Cephalhematoma occurs from rupture of small vessels in the periosteum. There is a soft swelling or lump, often the size and shape of a table tennis ball, with a very discrete edge (Figs. 37 and 38). They occur over the presenting part, usually the parietal bone, are sometimes bilateral and are often associated with caput. By contrast with caput, cephalhematomas are not apparent at birth, but there is a gradual ooze of blood from small vessel rupture, causing a slow increase to maximal size within a few days of birth. The swelling never crosses a suture.

Course and prognosis

They disappear spontaneously, sometimes accompanied by calcification, but may take several weeks or months to resolve completely. Jaundice is a common complication in the first few weeks.

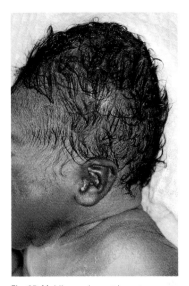

Fig. 35 Molding and caput in vertex presentation.

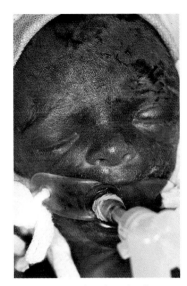

Fig. 36 Bruising of the face after face presentation.

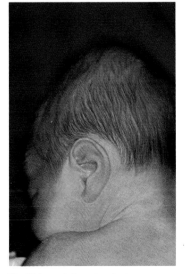

Fig. 37 Lateral view of parietal cephalhematoma.

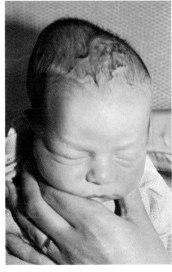

Fig. 38 Parietal cephalhematoma.

Facial palsy

Incidence | Common.

Etiology | Compression of the facial nerve as it exits from the parotid gland. The condition is sometimes caused by pressure from forceps blades but often occurs after normal vaginal delivery.

Clinical features | Weakness, usually unilateral, of the facial muscles (Fig. 39) that may cause drooping of the mouth (Fig. 40) and sometimes dribbling. There is often feeding difficulty and inability to close the eye on the affected side.

Prognosis | Majority resolve spontaneously within a few days or weeks after birth.

Erb's palsy

Incidence | Uncommon.

Etiology | Stretching or tearing of the upper part of the brachial plexus, usually caused by neck traction during breech delivery or with shoulder dystocia.

Clinical features | The affected arm and hand assume the waiter's tip position (Fig. 41)—weakness or paralysis of abduction at the shoulder, with flexion at the elbow and extension and supination of the wrist.

Prognosis | The weakness or paralysis usually responds spontaneously over a period of weeks or months, but paralysis is occasionally permanent. If resolution takes a long time, passive physiotherapy and night splints will prevent the formation of contractures.

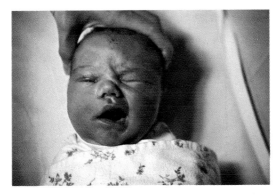

Fig. 39 Facial palsy after face presentation. Mouth is drawn down on the healthier side.

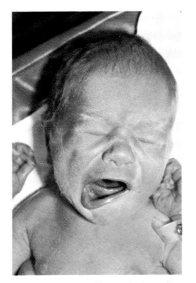

Fig. 40 Facial palsy affecting the lower lip.

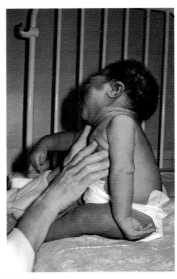

Fig. 41 Erb's palsy with arm in waiter's tip position.

Obstetric manipulations

Incidence

Obstetric manipulations often cause unavoidable, trivial skin trauma. With careful application and removal of instruments and equipment, they can usually be kept to a minimum.

Clinical features

Forceps application often results in pressure indentation or bruising (Fig. 42) and occasionally causes facial palsy or subcutaneous fat necrosis. Both of these complications can also occur after a spontaneous vaginal delivery, particularly after a long labor with slow descent of the presenting part. Subcutaneous fat necrosis can occur (Fig. 43) over any bony prominence but is most common on the cheek. It usually presents as an indurated, sometimes red, area that may then develop necrosis with loss of subcutaneous fat and sometimes calcification.

Artificial rupture of the membranes, fetal scalp sampling, and scalp electrodes may all cause incised wounds (Fig. 44). Particular care should be taken when removing scalp clips, as incorrect detachment may result in a core of scalp being removed.

Vacuum extraction, by applying suction to the scalp to assist delivery when there is delay in the second stage of labor, frequently causes bruising and a chignon-shaped caput. Sometimes it causes more serious blistering, abrasions, or laceration of the presenting part (Fig. 45) or occasionally subgaleal hemorrhage.

Significance

Lesions are usually trivial but may become the site of infection.

Course and prognosis

Most resolve spontaneously without significant scarring or more permanent sequelae.

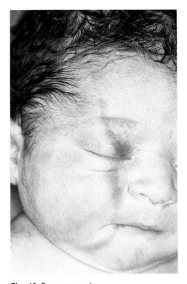

Fig. 42 Forceps mark.

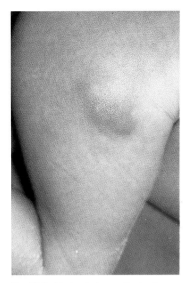

Fig. 43 Red indurated area of subcutaneous fat necrosis on thigh.

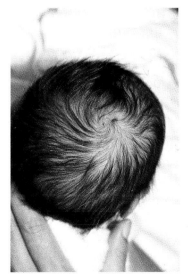

Fig. 44 Wound from a scalp clip used for fetal heart monitoring.

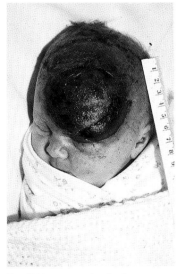

Fig. 45 Very severe abrasion from a prolonged application of vacuum.

3 / Deformations

Postural deformities

Incidence

Postural and compressional effects occur frequently. Most are mild and transient.

Clinical features

With abnormal presentations, the intrauterine posture is often maintained for several days after birth.

After a face or brow presentation, the infant may lie with head and neck extended in an opisthotonic posture.

After breech delivery, the head is not molded like that of a baby after vertex delivery. The legs are often maintained in hip flexion for some days (Figs. 46 and 47). In many normal infants, the feet are often molded into postural talipes (Fig. 48). Postural talipes can always be fully reduced by passive manipulation, and there is a full range of foot and ankle movement.

Extensive bruising of the presenting part often occurs, particularly if there has been an abnormal presentation. It resolves gradually over a few days and is often accompanied by hyperbilirubinemia.

Course and prognosis

After abnormal presentations, postural deformities disappear rapidly and spontaneously. Postural talipes may take months to resolve completely.

Management

No special management is required, as all improve spontaneously. Passive manipulation or even splinting of the feet is sometimes advised for postural talipes, but there is no evidence that it hastens normal resolution.

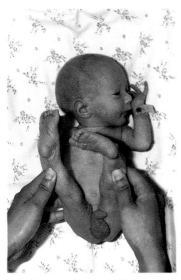

Fig. 46 Extended breech position.

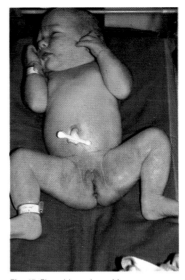

Fig. 47 Flexed breech position.

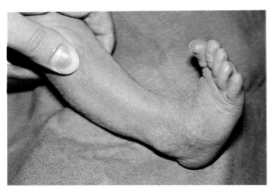

Fig. 48 Postural talipes.

4 / Iatrogenic lesions

Skin lesions

Incidence

With increasing use and complexity of neonatal intensive care, iatrogenic lesions, particularly of the skin, are becoming common.

Etiology and clinical features

Traumatic abrasions of the skin occur frequently, particularly in very preterm infants (Fig. 49) and may be associated with the use of adhesive tape, name bands, or starched sheets. Radiant heaters increase insensitive water loss through the transparent skin of preterm infants and may cause drying and fragility of the skin. Transcutaneous skin monitors for measuring O_2 and CO_2 always leave a transient, superficial, pink burn that does not usually cause scarring unless the electrode has been left in situ for a prolonged period. Depigmented circular areas of skin are sometimes seen later in dark-skinned infants (Fig. 50). Invasive procedures such as intercostal catheters for draining pneumothoraces (Fig. 51), radial artery puncture, and repeated heel pricking may leave scars. Intercostal catheters should be sited carefully, avoiding the area around the nipple to avoid more serious damage to the breast in later life.

Management and prevention

Measures should be taken to avoid excessive use of adhesive tape or equipment whenever possible. Protective covering may limit insensible water loss by evaporation in the days immediately after birth but will obviously depend on whether the clinical condition of the infant allows such covering. After the early days or weeks of life, the skin becomes much thicker and less prone to traumatic damage, even in very immature infants.

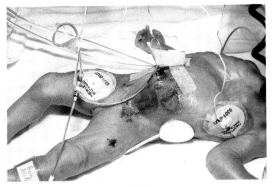

Fig. 49 Skin abrasions from adhesive tape.

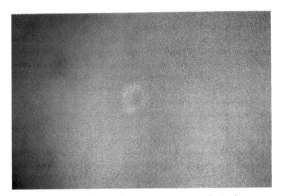

Fig. 50 Depigmented areas from transcutaneous electrode.

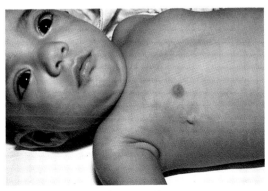

Fig. 51 Scar from a drain for pneumothorax.

Catheter and infusion complications

Clinical features and etiology

Catheters in major vessels may cause obstruction and ischemic necrosis to distal extremities, thrombosis, or embolism. Such complications are uncommon. Transient cyanosis of the leg is sometimes seen after insertion of an umbilical arterial catheter. If it does not resolve rapidly or if there is associated pallor or absence of arterial pulses, the catheter should be removed immediately. Cyanosis of the toes, particularly after arterial infusion is commenced, is not uncommon. It is usually transient and associated with minor air embolism.

With prolonged catheterization, the risk of infection and necrotizing enterocolitis increases. Peripheral intravenous infusion sites are often associated with edema or extravasation of the infusion fluid when the fluid extravasates into the subcutaneous tissue. Infusions containing irritants such as calcium or sodium bicarbonate may cause serious tissue necrosis (Fig. 52) and lead to ulceration and later scar formation (Figs. 53 and 54).

Management and prevention

Care should be taken in siting peripheral infusions to avoid veins near joints. Scarring around joints may cause contractures later. All intravenous drips should be checked frequently to ensure that they are running into the vein, particularly when infusion pumps are used. Central catheters should always be removed if there is persistent cyanosis of the extremities or if there are signs of catheter occlusion or impaired circulation to the limbs, kidneys, or gut. Arterial catheters should be removed as soon as the infant's clinical condition improves and when sampling for blood gas analysis is required less often.

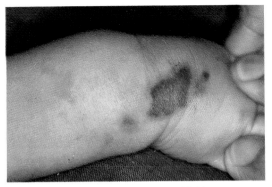

Fig. 52 Recent subcutaneous extravasation of fluid.

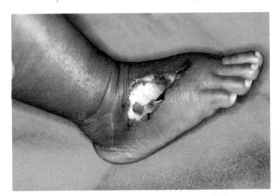

Fig. 53 Ulceration after extravasation of an irritant fluid.

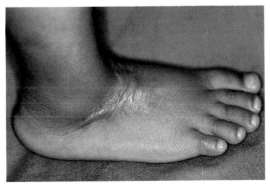

Fig. 54 Scar after an ulcer had healed.

5 / Skin disorders

Strawberry nevi

Incidence

Common, particularly in preterm infants.

Pathology

Dilated capillaries with or without endothelial proliferation.

Clinical features

Raised, soft, pitted, bright red hemangioma with a discrete edge. They are usually not present at birth but appear within the first few weeks of life. Hemangiomas are rarely seen in infants younger than 34 weeks postconceptional age. They are often preceded by a small and slightly raised, bright red spot, which evolves into the strawberry nevus (Fig. 55). They may be single or multiple and occur anywhere on the body.

Course and prognosis

Most increase rapidly in size during the first year of life. Ulceration and subsequent infection may occur in the center of the lesion. All strawberry nevi regress slowly over the next years. Involution has started when pale gray areas of fibrosis appear in the center of the nevus (Fig. 56). They eventually disappear completely (Fig. 57) and leave only a flat, pale depigmented area.

Management

No treatment is required, unless there is repeated hemorrhage, infection, or severe cosmetic deformity interfering with function of the affected part. All forms of treatment except steroids will leave some scarring of the skin; natural resolution is the optimal management in most strawberry nevi. When there is pressure on a vital organ or severe bleeding, steroids may sometimes be helpful.

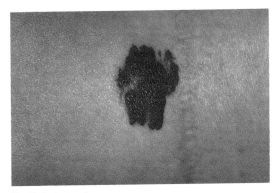

Fig. 55 Early strawberry nevus.

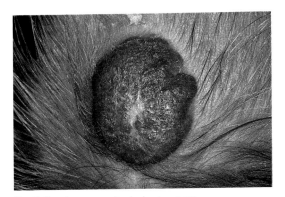

Fig. 56 Strawberry nevus beginning to regress.

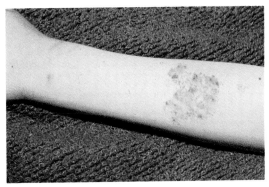

Fig. 57 Fading strawberry nevus.

Port wine stains

Synonym Nevus flammeus.

Clinical features Sharply demarcated flat capillary hemangioma that may vary in color from pale pink to deep purple (Fig. 58). They are present at birth and do not increase in size after birth. They may occur anywhere on the body but are most common on the face.

Course and prognosis Most remain as a permanent discoloration of the skin.

Associations Most port wine stains occur as an isolated defect but sometimes are partly cavernous, involve other organs, or form part of a recognizable vascular syndrome, e.g., Sturge–Weber syndrome (Fig. 59).

Management Generally, surgery is cosmetically unsatisfactory. The use of a cosmetic cover-up cream may be helpful in older children. Laser treatment is under investigation.

Cavernous hemangioma

Pathology Large, dilated blood-filled cavities with venous anastamoses. There is often a surface capillary element.

Clinical features Soft, subcutaneous bluish-red mass (Fig. 60) with a less distinct edge than a strawberry nevus.

Course and prognosis Most do not regress with age and may actually increase in size. Hemorrhage and infection sometimes occur, and occasionally sequestration of platelets within the nevus may cause thrombocytopenia.

Management Surgical excision is often difficult. Injection of sclerosing agents under anesthetic may promote fibrosis and eventual diminution in size.

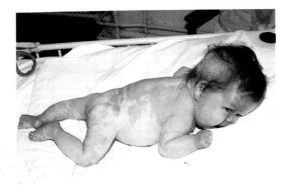

Fig. 58 Extensive port wine stain.

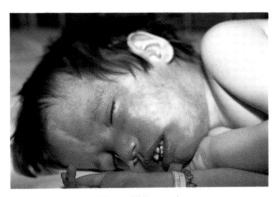

Fig. 59 Facial nevus of Sturge–Weber syndrome.

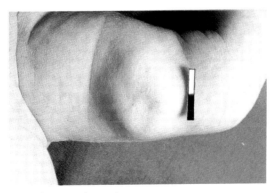

Fig. 60 Cavernous hemangioma.

Pigmented and depigmented nevi

Incidence

Uncommon in the neonatal period with the exception of Mongolian blue spots.

Clinical features

Small localized pigmented nevi are of no clinical significance. Severe cosmetic deformity may occur with the rare giant bathing trunk nevus. Incontinentia pigmenti, a rare sex-linked hereditary disorder, initially consists of inflammatory bullae in the neonatal period that progress to pigmented streaks in the later stages of the disease (Fig. 61)

Depigmented lesions are also uncommon and may occur as an isolated finding (Fig. 62). Occasionally, areas of skin or hair depigmentation may be the only manifestation of tuberose sclerosis in the neonatal period.

Management

Depends on the cosmetic deformity and presence or absence of associated disorders. Giant bathing trunk nevi are often grossly disfiguring and may be improved with multiple tiny skin grafts. Dermabrasion, if performed in the early weeks of life, may produce a major cosmetic improvement

Partial-thickness skin defects

Incidence

Rare

Etiology

Unknown.

Clinical features

The lesion is usually a superficial area of ulceration, most commonly found on the scalp.

Associations

Partial-thickness skin defects of the scalp sometimes occur in trisomy 13 (Patau syndrome Fig. 63).

Course and prognosis

The defect heals by granulation. If it is not superficial or if secondary infection occurs, healing may result in scar formation and contraction. A permanent bald patch may be left on the scalp.

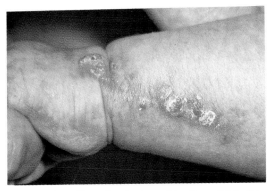

Fig. 61 Lesions of incontinentia pigmenti in a linear distribution.

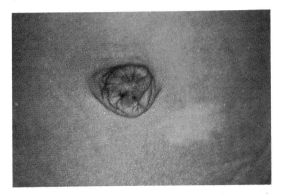

Fig. 62 Depigmented lesion alongside the umbilicus in a normal infant.

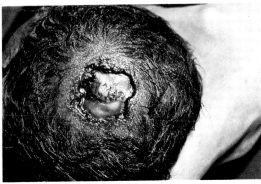

Fig. 63 Scalp skin defect in trisomy 13.

Epidermolysis bullosa letalis

Incidence

Very rare.

Inheritance

Autosomal recessive.

Pathology

Subepidermal bullae with blisters between the basement membrane of the epidermis and the connective tissue of the dermis.

Clinical features

Bullae present at or soon after birth and cover large areas of the body. Initial lesions commonly present at points of contact/pressure on the extensor surfaces. The bullae characteristically appear after minor trauma (Figs. 64 and 65).

Differential diagnosis

There are several different varieties of epidermolysis bullosa. Those that appear in later infancy are usually autosomal dominant and often dystrophic, resulting in scar formation. Epidermolysis bullosa may be similar in appearance to widespread staphylococcal skin infection (pemphigus neonatorum or toxic epidermal necrolysis) (Fig. 66) but should be differentiated by culture.

Management

Good nursing care is required, with particular emphasis on minimal handling because of the dramatic effect of minor trauma on the skin.

Antibiotics may be required if there is secondary bacterial infection.

Prognosis

High mortality in the neonatal form.

Antenatal diagnosis

A fetal skin biopsy in the second trimester may be helpful in high-risk pregnancies when there has been a previously affected infant.

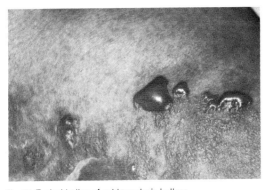

Fig. 64 Typical bullae of epidermolysis bullosa.

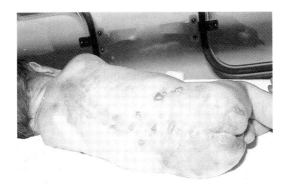

Fig. 65 Widespread bullae.

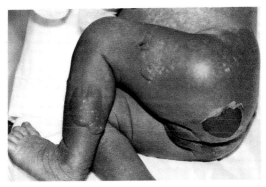

Fig. 66 Bullae may be similar in appearance to toxic epidermal necrolysis.

Collodion baby and harlequin fetus

Incidence   Very rare.

Etiology   Unknown.

Clinical features   At birth, the infant is encased in a shiny, brownish yellow, cellophane-like membrane (Figs. 67 and 68) that may be taut and may distort the facial features and extremities. Respiratory embarrassment may occur because of restriction of chest expansion. The much more severe condition called harlequin fetus has a similar appearance of the skin, but in addition there are deep fissures between scale-like areas of skin. Ectropion and everted lips (fish-mouth) also occur in the harlequin fetus. The harlequin vascular phenomenon is a quite different condition.

Course and prognosis   Desquamation of the membranous skin occurs after birth and may take several months to be complete. There is no particular treatment apart from the lubrication of the skin with creams (Fig. 69). The skin should not be allowed to become too dry, and secondary infection should be treated promptly. Prognosis should be guarded for collodion babies, because although most have normal skin in later childhood, a few develop ichthyotic skin changes later (Fig. 70). The harlequin fetus invariably dies in the neonatal period.

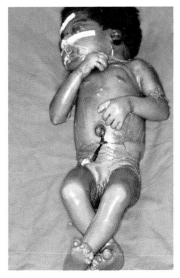

Fig. 67 Harlequin fetus.

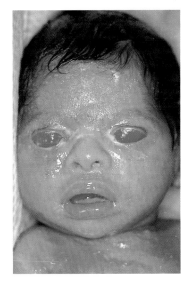

Fig. 68 Baby showing ectropion.

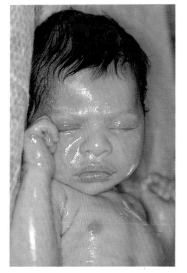

Fig. 69 Improvement is seen after 20 days. Note the oiled skin.

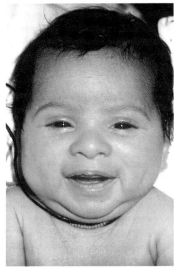

Fig. 70 Appearance of the baby in Figure 68 at 6 months. There was still some ichthyosis.

46

6 / Congenital abnormalities

Accessory skin tags and polydactyly

Incidence

Common, particularly in Afro-Caribbean infants.

Inheritance

Usually autosomal dominant.

Clinical features

Accessory skin tags (accessory auricles) often occur on the face, anterior to the ear (Fig. 71). Accessory nipples (Fig. 72) are often mistaken for pigmented nevi. They may be single or multiple and usually occur in a direct line beneath the normally situated nipple.

Extra digits (polydactyly) vary in appearance from loosely attached skin tags to fully formed fingers or toes (Fig. 73). They are usually attached at the base of the normal little finger or toe. Occasionally, there may be an associated bifid metacarpal or metatarsal bone.

Significance

Usually only a cosmetic deformity, but extra toes may cause broadening of the forefoot with difficulty in fitting shoes later.

Management

Small pedunculated tags can be ligated if the pedicle and base is very narrow and does not contain cartilage. The tag will become ischemic, but it is not painful. It will usually separate from the base within a few days, leaving a small dry scar. If the base is broad, or if the tag has a cartilaginous attachment, plastic surgery will be required.

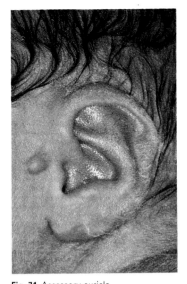

Fig. 71 Accessory auricle.

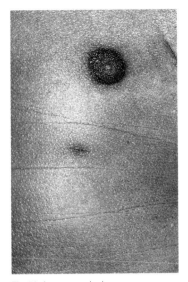

Fig. 72 Accessory nipple.

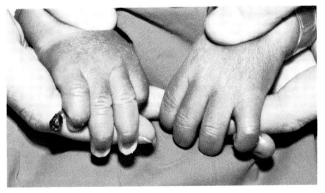

Fig. 73 Bilateral polydactyly.

Talipes equinovarus

Synonym

Club foot.

Incidence

Occurs in 1 in 1,000 live births. The condition is twice as common in males as in females.

Etiology

Uncertain; probably polygenic inheritance and intrauterine pressure play a part.

Clinical features

The affected foot is held in a fixed flexion (equinus) and inturned (varus) position (Fig. 74). It can be differentiated from positional talipes because the deformity in true talipes cannot be passively corrected.

Associations

Usually occurs as an isolated deformity but may occur in association with meningomyelocele, oligohydramnios, and congenital dislocation of the hip.

Management

Correction of the deformity is usually initially attempted by splinting, but if correction is difficult, surgical release of the contracted structures in the calf and ankle may be necessary.

Toe deformities

Incidence

Common—particularly syndactyly.

Inheritance

Mostly autosomal dominant.

Clinical features

Syndactyly usually occurs as webbing of the second and third toes.
Overlapping of the little toe over the fourth toe is usually bilateral (Fig. 75). Hammer toe usually occurs in the big toe and results from a congenital contracture of the flexor tendons (Fig. 76).

Management

Syndactyly of toes does not require surgery. The position of the toes in hammer toe or overlapping little toe is usually uncomfortable, and surgical correction may be needed.

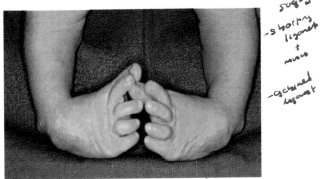

sugg
-shorting
ligaret
+
muscle
-achieved
ligaret

Fig. 74 Bilateral talipes equinovarus.

sole
-inverted medially

Metatarsus varus

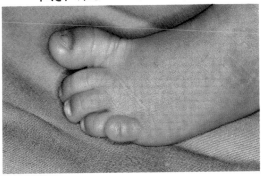

Fig. 75 Overriding little toe.

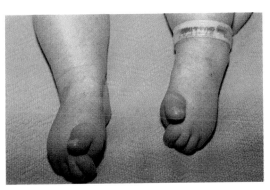

Fig. 76 Bilateral hammer toes.

Neural tube defects (1)

Meningomyelocele, spina bifida; encephalocele; anencephaly.

Incidence
Varies in different geographic locations. It is particularly common in the United States and United Kingdom, where the overall incidence of neural tube defects is 1 in 300 pregnancies. Neural tube defects are more common in the Welsh and Irish than in the English. The high birth prevalence is falling for reasons that are not yet clear but may be related to antenatal screening with ultrasound and alphafetoprotein and improved maternal nutrition. Spina bifida occulta occurs in at least 1% of the normal population.

Etiology
Unknown but maternal folic acid supplements taken around the time of conception have been shown to reduce the incidence of neural tube defects in high-risk families.

Inheritance
Polygenic. After one affected child, there is a 1 in 20 risk of recurrence of a neural tube defect in the next pregnancy.

Antenatal diagnosis
Elevated alphafetoprotein concentrations in amniotic fluid and maternal plasma occur in the second trimester of pregnancy in most open neural tube defects. Spinal defects are usually apparent on ultrasound examination.

Clinical features

Meningomyelocele and meningocele
A fluid-filled sac often containing neural tissue (meningomyelocele), with an underlying defect of the spinal arch, occurs in the lumbosacral region (Figs. 77 & 78) in 94% of cases. The degree of handicap depends on the level and severity of the defect. There may be flaccid paralysis of the lower limbs, sensory loss, a neurogenic bladder with urinary incontinence, and a patulous anus (Fig. 79) with fecal incontinence. Meningoceles often occur in the thoracic (Fig. 80) or cervical spine. ➡

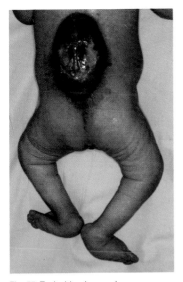

Fig. 77 Typical lumbosacral meningomyelocele.

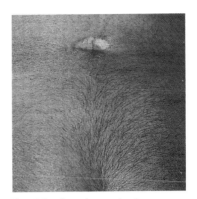

Fig. 78 Small meningomyelocele.

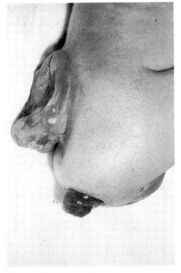

Fig. 79 Meningomyelocele with paralyzed anus. There is a rectal prolapse.

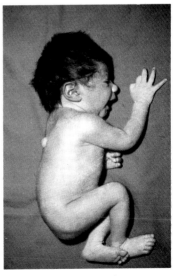

Fig. 80 Thoracic meningocele.

Neural tube defects (2)

Associations Hydrocephalus occurs in 70% of cases of meningomyelocele. Congenital dislocation of the hip and talipes equinovarus are common. Urinary tract infections often occur.

Management Surgery may be indicated in less severely handicapped infants after careful assessment of the congenital abnormalities and neurologic state of the infant in the first few days of life. Skin closure is the first operation, but many other surgical procedures may be required to treat hydrocephalus, and orthopedic and urinary problems. The meningoceles in the thoracic or cervical regions usually have an excellent prognosis as there are no associated neurologic abnormalities.

Encephalocele

Clinical features Herniation of the meninges and brain through the skull (Fig. 81).

Course and prognosis Depends on the amount of brain that has to be excised to close the skull defect, but the prognosis is not necessarily poor. The lesions are usually occipital.

Anencephaly

Clinical features Absence of the forebrain and skull vault, and secondary distortion of the face and ears (Fig. 82).

Associations Other abnormalities are common, particularly cleft palate and abnormal cervical vertebrae. It is more common in females.

Course and prognosis Anencephaly is incompatible with life. Many infants are stillborn, although a few may survive for several hours and occasionally days.

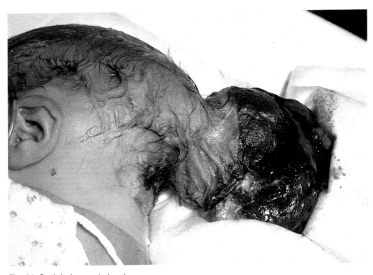

Fig. 81 Occipital encephalocele.

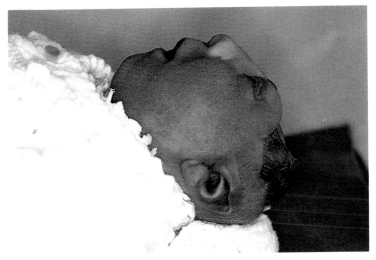

Fig. 82 Anencephaly—a postmortem photograph.

Hydrocephalus

Etiology

May occur as an isolated congenital abnormality. The condition is most commonly due to aqueduct stenosis or secondary to intraventricular hemorrhage or neonatal meningitis. It is commonly found in association with neural tube defects.

Clinical features

Accelerated rate of growth of the skull gives rise to enlargement of the head circumference (Fig. 83), widening of the fontanelles and sutures. When severe and untreated, hydrocephalus may give rise to a setting-sun appearance of the eyes, mental handicap and upper motor neuron signs, particularly in the legs.

Management

Depends on etiology and severity. Ultrasound and computed tomography scan will confirm the diagnosis. If there is evidence of continuing deviation from the normal rate of growth of the ventricles or skull circumference, a ventriculoperitoneal or ventriculoatrial shunt may be required.

Course and prognosis

Not all infants with hydrocephalus require neurosurgery. After intraventricular hemorrhage, hydrocephalus may be transient and limited by serial lumbar puncture. After shunt surgery, the prognosis depends on the underlying etiology, extent of preceding brain damage, and the occurrence of shunt complications.

Microcephaly

Clinical features

Head circumference below the 3rd centile for age and gestation (Fig. 84) and inappropriately small for the length and weight of the infant.

Etiology

Usually unknown; often associated with mental retardation. Sometimes a clear prenatal cause is known, e.g., congenital rubella or cytomegalovirus infection.

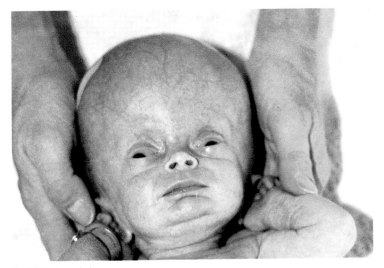

Fig. 83 Hydrocephalus.

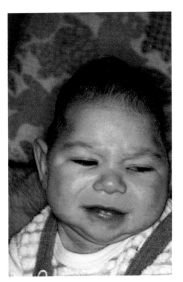

Fig. 84 Microcephaly at 11 months of age.

Cleft lip and palate

Incidence Common; approximately 1 in 600 live births. It is more frequent in East Asia.

Inheritance Familial. There is no simple mendelian pattern. Inheritance is probably polygenic.

Clinical features Isolated clefts of the palate always occur in the midline. The least obvious type is the submucous cleft, which is often associated with a bifid uvula. Cleft lip and palate may be unilateral (Fig. 85) or bilateral.

Associations Feeding difficulties and orthodontic deformities are common. Speech problems may occur with cleft palate, particularly after late closure. Deafness may arise secondary to regurgitation and sepsis in the nasopharynx.

Management Some infants can feed from the breast; most infants feed well through a large nipple. Tube or spoon feeding may occasionally be needed. Surgery is performed in several stages. Repair of the cleft lip to correct the cosmetic deformity should be performed as soon as possible after birth. The palate repair is usually performed later, but within the first year of life an excellent cosmetic result is usually achieved (Figs. 86 and 87). If the initial deformity is severe, secondary repair of the lip or nose or pharyngoplasty may be required in later childhood.

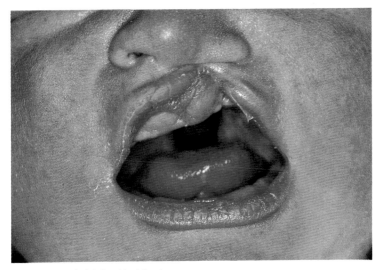

Fig. 85 Unilateral cleft lip with cleft palate.

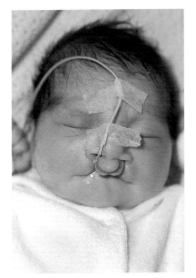

Fig. 86 Cleft lip and palate.

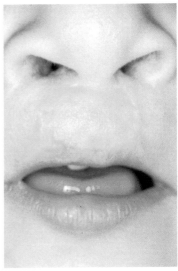

Fig. 87 Same patient in Figure 86 at 4 years of age, after surgery.

Cataracts

Incidence

Uncommon.

Etiology

Congenital cataracts are often inherited as an autosomal dominant. They may also occur secondary to intrauterine infections, particularly rubella, or metabolic disorders such as galactosemia.

Clinical features

An opaque mass can be seen in the pupil (Fig. 88).

Management

Depends on the type and severity of the cataract and the interference with vision. Metabolic disorders, which may be potentially treatable, should always be excluded. Early surgery is indicated within the first month of life in those cataracts that warrant treatment. After surgery for cataracts at any age, contact lenses will need to be fitted and replaced at regular intervals.

Cystic hygroma

Incidence

Uncommon.

Etiology

Hamartoma of the jugular lymphatic vessels.

Clinical features

Soft, multicystic, and ill-defined fluctuant lymphatic swelling in the lateral part of the neck (Fig. 89). The cysts transilluminate well and enlarge slowly during the first few months or years of life. The effect on the child depends on the size and site of the abnormality but can occasionally cause dysphagia or respiratory obstruction, particularly if it enlarges rapidly. Occasionally, enlargement may be due to infection or hemorrhage.

Management

Surgical excision is difficult because of the invasive, ill-defined nature of the lymphatic channels, but it is usually necessary.

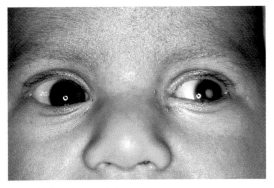

Fig. 88 Unilateral congenital cataract.

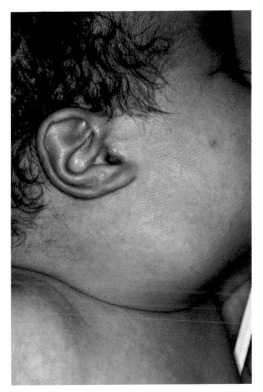

Fig. 89 Cystic hygroma.

Congenital dislocation of the hip

Incidence

Dislocated or dislocatable hip at birth may be as common as 1 in 100 live births. With early detection and treatment, the prevalence of dislocated hip after the first year of life has been reduced from 1:1,000 to 1:10,000. It is more common in girls and after breech presentation.

Inheritance

Familial. There is no simple mendelian pattern of inheritance.

Clinical features

Most should be detected by routine screening tests in the neonatal period. Fixed dislocation can be diagnosed by finding restricted abduction of the hip and sometimes shortening of the affected leg.

To examine for a reducible dislocation, the infant should be placed on its back on a firm surface. Holding the thighs between finger and thumb with the hips and knees both flexed, each hip should be slowly abducted through 90° starting from the midline (Figs. 90–92). A palpable "clunk" will be felt as a posteriorly dislocated hip slips back into the acetabulum. A gentle attempt should then be made to diagnose a dislocatable hip. With the leg adducted, pressure is applied with the thumb on the upper part of the femur; the leg is then abducted, as above. Ultrasound is becoming useful in diagnosis and may be used as a screening procedure in the future.

Management

Abduction splinting is required for at least 6 weeks. Even a dislocatable hip that resolves spontaneously should be observed until the child is walking. X-ray all hips where neonatal examinations have aroused suspicion at 4–6 months of age. Delay in diagnosis may involve more prolonged splinting or surgery. With early diagnosis and treatment, most infants with congenital dislocation of the hip should have no delay in crawling or walking.

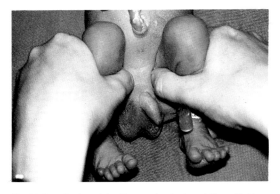

Fig. 90 Examination of the hips starting in the midline with hips and knees flexed.

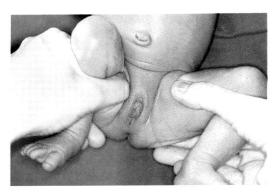

Fig. 91 Abduction of the hip holding the thigh between fingers and thumb.

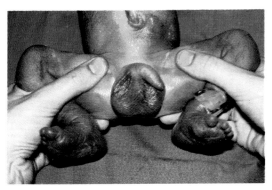

Fig. 92 Full abduction of both hips through 90°.

Congenital heart disease

Incidence

Occurs in 7 in 1,000 live births. There is a high incidence in infants of diabetic mothers and infants with chromosomal abnormalities.

Clinical features

Most present with a heart murmur, cardiac failure, or cyanosis (Fig. 93). They may become breathless and sweat with feeding and usually fail to thrive.

Management

Careful clinical examination, including blood pressure and electrocardiograph, may be helpful in the assessment. Echocardiography is the most useful diagnostic procedure.

Esophageal atresia and tracheoesophageal fistula

Incidence

Occurs in 1 in 3,000 live births; often occurs with other congenital abnormalities.

Clinical features

Excessive accumulation of saliva and mucus in the mouth and pharynx occurs because there is a developmental anomaly with a blind-ending upper esophageal pouch. There is a high incidence of associated duodenal atresia; cardiac, renal, and skeletal defects may also be associated. Imperforate anus may be associated. Respiratory distress may occur if there is spillover into the trachea or regurgitation of stomach contents through a fistula. Pulmonary complications frequently occur if the baby is fed before the diagnosis is suspected.

Diagnosis

Maternal hydramnios occurs in 60% of babies with esophageal atresia. The atresia is now often diagnosed by antenatal ultrasound. Whenever atresia is suspected, a firm catheter should be passed to test for gastric acid. Chest radiograph will usually confirm esophageal atresia (Fig. 94). Air in the stomach indicates the presence of a fistula.

Management

Arrange for delivery in a perinatal center with a pediatric surgical service. Early surgery with primary anastamosis is indicated if possible. Fistulas should be sought and ligated.

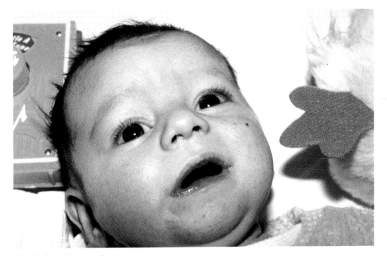

Fig. 93 Central cyanosis.

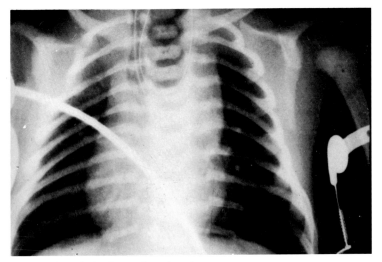

Fig. 94 Radiograph showing esophageal atresia.

Amniotic bands and amputations

Incidence

Uncommon, but exact incidence is not known. Clustering of cases has been reported.

Etiology

Unknown. The most widely accepted hypothesis suggests that the developing embryo may lie in a false cavity between the amnion and chorion after traumatic rupture of the manion in the first trimester. The membranes may then form encircling bands around the limbs. An alternative hypothesis is that vascular occlusion secondary to embolization from thrombosed placental vessels may cause the abnormalities.

Associations

Amniotic bands may be associated with fetal malformations, particularly limb or craniofacial defects.

Clinical features

The presence of amniotic bands is usually inferred when constriction rings (Fig. 95) or reduction deformities of the limbs occur (Fig. 96). Occasionally, a band may be attached to the fetus at the site of a local abnormality.

Limb reduction deformities

Etiology

A famous outbreak in the early 1960s was due to the effects of a teratogen—thalidomide. Many cases occur without any known cause.

Clinical features

The lesion is obvious at birth (Fig. 97). The limb is short, and a rudimentary hand or foot may be attached to the shoulder or hip.

Management

A search should be made for other abnormalities. The baby is referred to a limb-fitting center in early life.

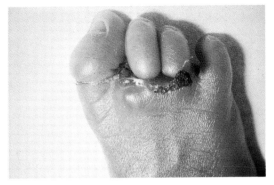

Fig. 95 Constriction ring around toes.

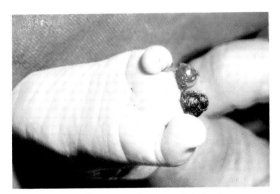

Fig. 96 Gangrene of toes secondary to amniotic bands.

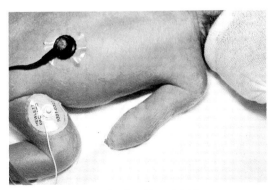

Fig. 97 Arm reduction deformity with vestigial fingers.

Down syndrome

Synonyms

Trisomy 21; used to be called mongolism.

Incidence

Occurs in 1 in 600 live births. It is the most common chromosomal abnormality.

Inheritance

Increased incidence of trisomy 21 with older maternal age (1 in 100 live births after maternal age of 40 years and 1 in 50 after 45 years). General risk of recurrence is 1% but may be higher if there is translocation and, for older mothers, is the expected incidence for maternal age.

Etiology

Trisomy 21 occurs in 94%, translocation in 3%, and mosaicism in 3%.

Clinical features

Low birth weight and growth retardation are common. Mongoloid facies (Figs. 98 and 99), generalized hypotonia, brachycephaly with a flattened occiput, a third fontanelle, and single transverse palmar creases (Simian crease, Fig. 100) are usually present. There may also be incurving of short fifth finger, a wide gap between second and third toe, marked plantar crease, congenital heart disease, and Brushfield spots.

[handwritten margin notes:]
- loose ears
- nuchal folds
- protrusia of tongue
- micrographia

[handwritten note:] AV canal / VSD / ASD

Associations

Increased incidence of respiratory infection, leukemia, thyroid disease, duodenal atresia, and Hirschsprung's disease.

Course and prognosis

Short stature and mental retardation are always present. Average IQ is <50, although social performance is often beyond that expected for mental age. Males are invariably infertile, but females are not necessarily so. Average life span is 30–40 years.

Antenatal diagnosis

Amniocentesis and chromosomal analysis may be indicated in older mothers or when there has been a previously affected child and when there is a translocation. A combination of biochemical tests is being used to identify women at high risk.

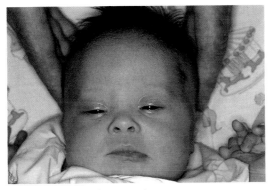

Fig. 98 Typical facies of Down syndrome.

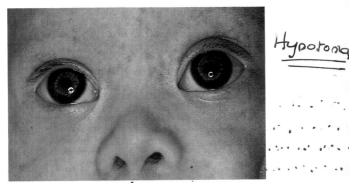

Hypotonia

Fig. 99 Prominent epicanthic folds in Down syndrome. Note Brushfield spots on the iris.

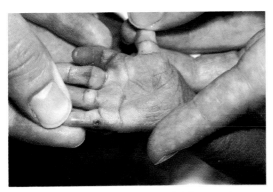

Fig. 100 Single transverse palmar crease (Simian crease).

Edward syndrome

Synonyms Trisomy 18, E-trisomy.

Incidence Occurs in 1 in 3,000 live births. It is the second most common chromosomal abnormality.

Inheritance Recurrence risk is low.

Clinical features
- Small for gestational age.
- Severe mental retardation.
- Hypoplastic lungs.
- Congenital heart disease.
- Abnormal posture with flexion deformities of hips and limbs (Fig. 101).
- Clenched hands with overlapping of index finger over third, and fifth finger over fourth finger (Fig. 102).
- Rocker-bottom feet (Fig. 103).
- Renal abnormalities and cryptorchidism.
- Craniofacial abnormalities with prominent occiput, micrognathia, hirsutism, short palpebral fissures, microstomia, facial palsy, and low-set ears.
- Hypoplasia of nails.

Course and prognosis Majority die within the first few months of life. Less than 10% survive longer than 1 year.

Patau syndrome

Synonyms Trisomy 13, D-trisomy.

Inheritance Recurrence risk is low.

Clinical features
- Midline defects of face, eyes and forebrain.
- Cleft lip and palate.
- Severe mental retardation.
- Deafness.
- Rocker-bottom feet (Fig. 103).
- Congenital heart defects.
- Cryptorchidism.
- Cutis aplasia.
- Polydactyly.
- Prominent heels.

Course and prognosis Less than 20% survive the first year of life.

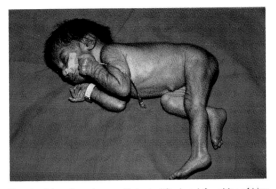

Fig. 101 Edward syndrome with typical flexion deformities of hips and limbs.

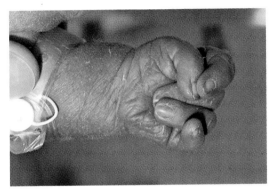

Fig. 102 Clenched hands with overlapping of fingers in Edward syndrome.

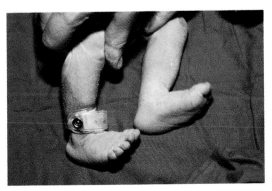

Fig. 103 Rocker-bottom feet.

Turner syndrome

Synonyms	XO syndrome, single X syndrome.
Incidence	Occurs in 1 in 5,000 live births.
Inheritance	Usually sporadic occurrence.
Etiology	Premature ovarian failure. Single X chromosome and absence of sex chromatin.
Clinical features	Low-birth-weight female infants with transient congenital lymphedema of hands and feet (Fig. 104). There is also webbing of the neck, broad chest with widely spaced nipples, low hairline and short neck, and a wide carrying angle (cubitus valgus).
Associations	Coarctation of aorta, deafness, and mild mental deficiency occur in about 10%.
Course and prognosis	Short stature and failure of secondary sexual development become apparent in later childhood.
Management	Cyclical estrogen replacement therapy will be indicated during adolescence and adult life to induce development of secondary sexual characteristics. Infertility is invariable.

Short-limbed dwarfism

Synonym	Chondrodysplasia.
Incidence	Achondroplasia, the most common chondrodysplasia, occurs in 1 in 10,000 live births.
Inheritance	Autosomal dominant inheritance; approximately 90% occur as a fresh mutation. The lethal forms of chondrodysplasia (asphyxiating thoracic dystrophy or thanatophoric dwarfism) are usually autosomal recessive (Fig. 105).
Clinical features	Short limbs, a large head (macrocephaly), and a prominent forehead with a broad nasal bridge.
Course and prognosis	Intelligence is usually normal in achondroplastic dwarfs, but early motor development is slow.

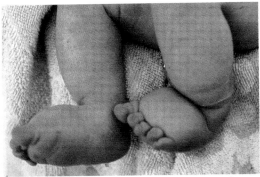

Fig. 104 Lymphedema of feet in Turner syndrome.

- hypoplasic
- oedema
- primary prepern
- nearby/b

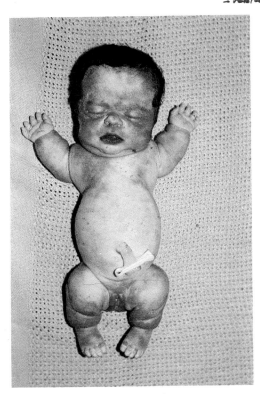

Fig. 105 Asphyxiating thoracic dystrophy.

Potter syndrome

Synonym — Renal agenesis.

Incidence — Occurs in 1 in 3,000 live births.

Etiology — The classic syndrome described by Potter was due to renal agenesis of unknown etiology. Other renal defects (polycystic kidneys or chronic urinary tract obstruction) or chronic leakage of amniotic fluid may also give rise to oligohydramnios and similar clinical manifestations.

Inheritance — Sporadic occurrence.

Clinical features

* cleft
* micrognathia

- Low birth weight.
- Low-set ears (Fig. 106).
- Compression abnormalities with flexion contractures of limbs.
- Hypoplastic lungs.
- Renal failure.

Course and prognosis — Renal insufficiency and progressive biochemical derangement occur. Death is normally due to respiratory failure soon after birth.

Prune-belly syndrome

Incidence — Uncommon.

Inheritance — Sporadic occurrence.

Clinical features

- Deficient abdominal wall musculature giving a rugose, prune-belly appearance (Fig. 107).
- Undescended testis.
- Multiple renal abnormalities.

Management — Surgical management of renal abnormalities if appropriate. Reconstitution of abdominal wall at a later stage.

Prognosis — Depends on the severity of renal abnormalities.

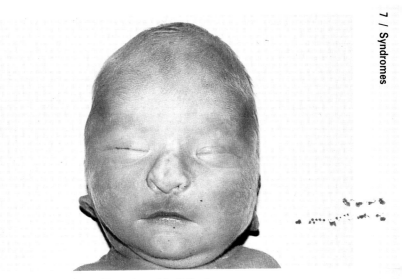

Fig. 106 Potter syndrome. (By courtesy of Dr. G. Gau.)

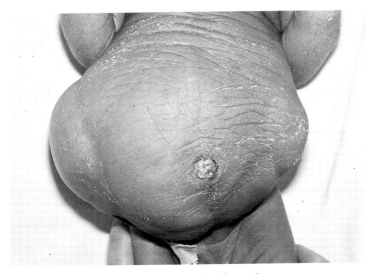

Fig. 107 Prune-belly syndrome with lax abdominal wall musculature.

Androgenital syndrome

Synonym	Congenital adrenal hyperplasia.
Incidence	Occurs in 1 in 5,000 for 21-hydroxylase deficiency. The other enzyme defects are much rarer.
Etiology	This group of disorders is caused by absence of essential enzymes in the pathway of cortisol and aldosterone synthesis. As a result, there is androgen excess. The most common variety is due to 21-hydroxylase deficiency.
Inheritance	Autosomal recessive.
Clinical features	Affected females are virilized at birth and may be confused for males with hypospadias and cryptorchidism (Figs. 108 and 109). Male infants may not be diagnosed until they develop an adrenal crisis in the second week of life, with vomiting and weight loss.
Investigation	A salt-losing adrenal crisis will be associated with hyponatremia and hyperkalemia. Grossly elevated serum 17-hydroxyprogesterone suggests the diagnosis of 21-hydroxylase deficiency. Elevated urinary pregnanetriol and 17-oxosteroids will confirm the diagnosis. Antenatal diagnosis is possible, and neonatal screening has been proposed.
Management	Urgent intravenous saline will be required to treat a severe salt-losing crisis. The aim of long-term management is to suppress the hyperplastic adrenal glands and to provide physiologic replacement of glucocorticoids and mineralocorticoids with hydrocortisone and fludrocortisone. The masculinized female infant may require plastic surgery in early childhood.
Prognosis	Correct replacement therapy will ensure normal linear growth. Hydrocortisone and fludrocortisone replacement is required for life.

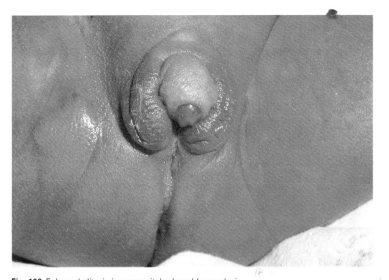

Fig. 108 Enlarged clitoris in congenital adrenal hyperplasia.

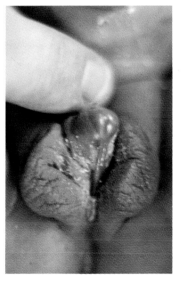

Fig. 109 Enlarged clitoris and rugose labia majora, which could be confused with severe hypospadias.

Osteogenesis imperfecta

Synonym	Brittle bone disease.
Incidence	Uncommon.
Inheritance	The severe congenital broad-boned type of osteogenesis imperfecta is usually autosomal recessive. Other less severe forms may be autosomal dominant.
Etiology	Unknown. There appears to be an abnormality of collagen formation.
Clinical features	Poorly mineralized skull and long bones with multiple fractures and callus formation. In the severe form, they often have short, deformed limbs at birth due to intrauterine fractures (Figs. 110 and 111). Crepitus may be felt in bones with recent fractures. Blue sclerae are sometimes present but may be difficult to diagnose in the neonatal period.
Prognosis	There is wide variability in the natural history of the disorder, with stillbirth or early mortality among severely affected infants. Beyond infancy, the outlook for survival is good, but the child is often handicapped by orthopedic deformity and deafness secondary to otosclerosis.
Management	Careful nursing is mandatory. Orthopedic treatment of fractures is the only form of treatment that can be offered, but optimal management will limit deformity.

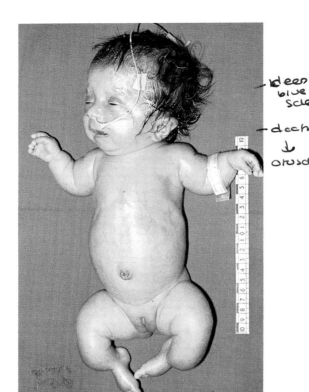

deep
blue
sclera

dentin
↓
osteodentin

Fig. 110 Osteogenesis imperfecta.

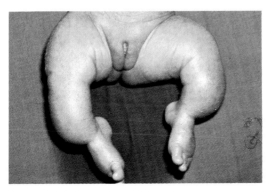

Fig. 111 Legs of a baby who had intrauterine fractures from osteogenesis imperfecta.

Congenital hypothyroidism

Synonym Cretinism.

Incidence Occurs in 1 in 6,000 live births.

Etiology Defective thyroid gland development, occasionally secondary to maternal goitrogens or inborn errors of thyroxine synthesis.

Clinical features
- Coarse facies and large protruding tongue (Figs. 112 and 113).
- Hoarse cry.
- Poor weight gain.
- Umbilical hernia (Figs. 113 and 114).
- Constipation.
- Prolonged jaundice.
- Hypothermia.
- Absence of spontaneous activity and crying.
- Feeding difficulties.

Associations Rarely, a goiter may occur when hypothyroidism is secondary to maternal goitrogens or an inborn error of thyroxine synthesis.

Management Thyroid hormone replacement for life.

Prognosis Early diagnosis and treatment within 2 months of birth improves the outlook for normal mental development in most cases. Routine screening of all infants within a few days of birth now ensures early diagnosis and treatment. This may reduce morbidity, but there is still some reduction in intellectual and motor functions.

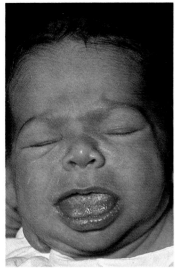

Fig. 112 Coarse facies and large protruding tongue of congenital hypothyroidism.

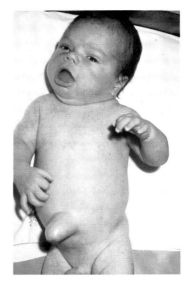

Fig. 113 Umbilical hernia and large tongue.

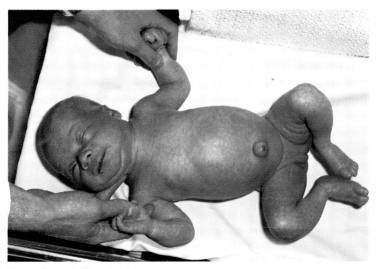

Fig. 114 Congenital hypothyroidism.

Pierre Robin syndrome

Synonym	Robin anomalad.
Incidence	Relatively common.
Inheritance	Usually sporadic occurrence.
Etiology	Early developmental anomaly with mandibular hypoplasia, posterior location of the tongue, and impaired closure of the posterior palate.
Clinical features	Severe micrognathia (Fig. 115). Wide posterior midline cleft palate (Fig. 116).
Complications	Acute respiratory obstruction because of a tendency of the tongue to fall back into the cleft palate; feeding difficulties.
Management	Expert nursing is required, often with the infant in the face-down posture to prevent respiratory obstruction. Surgical closure of the cleft palate should be performed after 3 months of age.
Course and prognosis	High mortality in early infancy due to acute respiratory obstruction. Micrognathia and glossoptosis improve during infancy.

Klippel–Feil syndrome

Incidence	Occurs in about 1 in 40,000 live births. There is a female predominance.
Inheritance	Sporadic occurrence of unknown etiology.
Clinical features	There is a short immobile neck, secondary webbing of neck, low hairline (Fig. 117), and fusion of cervical vertebrae. Hemivertebrae, rib defects, scoliosis, and Sprengel's shoulder sometimes occur. There may also be secondary torticollis and facial asymmetry.
Associations	Deafness in approximately 30% of cases. The syndrome may occur as part of a more serious defect of neural tube development.

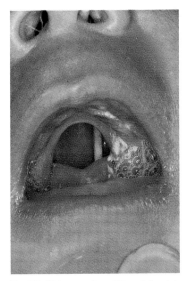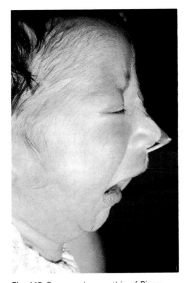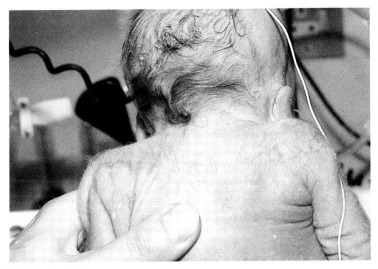

Fig. 115 Severe micrognathia of Pierre Robin syndrome.

Fig. 116 Wide posterior midline cleft palate.

Fig. 117 Short neck and low hairline in Klippel–Feil syndrome.

☘ Infant of diabetic mother

Incidence

Good control of maternal diabetes throughout pregnancy reduces the signs and symptoms in infants of diabetic mothers, except the increased risk of congenital abnormalities.

Clinical features

Large obese infants (Figs. 118 and 119) who are at higher risk for developing respiratory distress syndrome close to term and are at significant risk for traumatic birth injury. After birth, there is a risk of hypoglycemia due to islet cell hyperplasia, and of polycythemia.

Management

Infants of diabetic mothers require careful observation in the first few hours after birth, with regular monitoring of blood sugar. Hypoglycemia usually responds to frequent milk feedings or an intravenous infusion of dextrose.

Course and prognosis

The hypoglycemia settles within a few days and, provided it has been recognized and treated adequately, will not give rise to any sequelae. These infants may have other electrolyte abnormalities, particularly hypocalcemia and hypomagnesemia.

Prevention

The frequency of congenital abnormalities (5%) is higher than the general population risk (3%). It is not yet known whether meticulous diabetic control before conception will reduce this high risk.

Beckwith–Wiedemann syndrome

Incidence

Rare.

Etiology

Unknown.

Inheritance

Usually sporadic occurrence.

Clinical features

Large-birth-weight infants with glossoptosis (Fig. 120) and omphalocele. Hypoglycemia due to pancreatic hyperplasia and polycythemia often occur.

Prognosis

High mortality in the neonatal period.

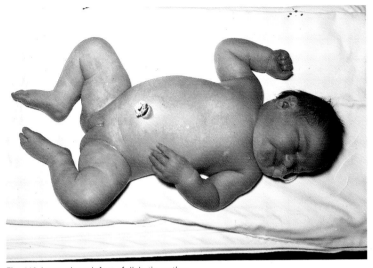

Fig. 118 Large obese infant of diabetic mother.

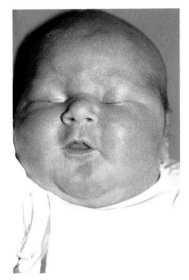

Fig. 119 Cherubic facies of infant of diabetic mother.

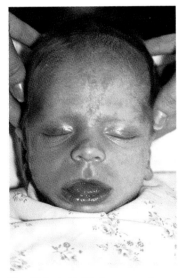

Fig. 120 Beckwith–Wiedemann syndrome with glossoptosis.

Hydrops fetalis

Incidence

Uncommon; less common since the prevention of rhesus disease with anti-D.

Etiology

- Hemolytic disease, particularly rhesus isoimmunization or other major antigen incompatibilities (e.g., anti-C, anti-E). ABD incompatibility does not cause hydrops.
- α-Thalassemia.
- Intrauterine viral infections, particularly cytomegalovirus.
- Congenital syphilis.
- Supraventricular tachycardia with congestive cardiac failure.
- Congenital nephrotic syndrome.
- Congenital parvovirus infection.
- Placental angioma.
- Chromosomal disorders (e.g. trisomy 21, Turner syndrome).

Clinical features

- Pallor.
- Gross generalized edema (Figs. 121 and 122).
- Ascites.
- Pleural effusions.
- Congestive heart failure.
- Severe respiratory distress due to pulmonary edema or pulmonary hypoplasia.

Management

Depends on the cause of hydrops. If hydrops is secondary to hemolytic disease, exchange transfusions and ventilatory support are the mainstay of treatment.

In the presence of cardiac failure secondary to a tachyarrhythmia, treatment is directed toward correcting the arrhythmia with drugs or defibrillation and supportive treatment of cardiac failure.

Prognosis

Depends on the underlying cause. The prognosis is usually good if the infant survives the neonatal period.

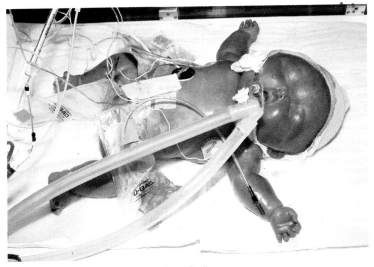

Fig. 121 Gross generalized edema of hydrops fetalis.

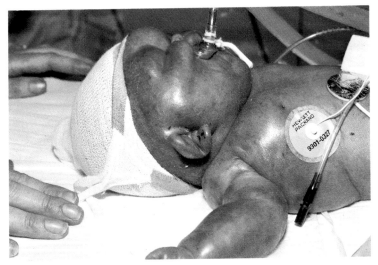

Fig. 122 Pallor and edema in hydrops fetalis due to rhesus hemolytic disease.

Staphylococcal infection

Incidence

Serious staphylococcal infection is now uncommon, but minor superficial infections are not.

Etiology

Bacterial infection caused by Gram-positive cocci, *Staphylococcus aureus*. Some strains of this bacterium produce a toxin called exfoliatin.

Clinical features

Superficial staphylococcal infections result in small pustules anywhere on the skin (Figs. 123 and 124). Umbilical sepsis (Fig. 125) is very common, and if there is a frank discharge or periumbilical cellulitis, systemic antibiotics will be required. Paronychia of the fingers and toes, although apparently minor infections, may cause more serious sepsis if not promptly treated. Occasionally, toxic epidermal necrolysis (TEN, scalded skin syndrome, or Ritter disease) with extensive X epidermal separation may develop (Fig. 126).

Complications

Septicemia, meningitis, and osteomyelitis.

Management

All superficial infections in young infants should be promptly treated with broad-spectrum systemic antibiotics after appropriate swabs and cultures.

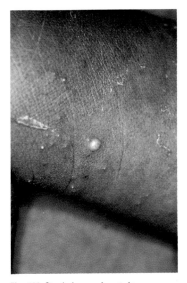

Fig. 123 Staphylococcal pustule.

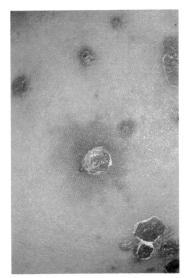

Fig. 124 Impetiginous staphylococcal lesions.

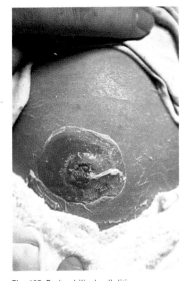

Fig. 125 Periumbilical cellulitis.

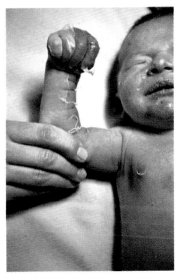

Fig. 126 Toxic epidermal necrolysis.

Neonatal ophthalmia

Incidence	Minor sticky eye is extremely common.
Etiology	Conjunctivitis may be due to a variety of organisms, the most serious being the sexually transmitted *Neiserria gonorrhoea* and *Chlamydia trachomatis*.
Clinical features	Manifestations vary from a mild sticky eye (Fig. 127) to severe conjunctival inflammation with a purulent discharge and periorbital edema. Gonococcal ophthalmia causes severe signs within 48 h of birth (Fig. 128). Chlamydia infection (Fig. 129) often does not become apparent until the second week of life and may coexist with gonorrhea.
Diagnosis	Appropriate swabs should be taken, but treatment should be commenced immediately if gonorrhea is suspected.
Management	Minor sticky eyes are usually noninfective and respond to saline eye washes. Gonococcal ophthalmia should be treated with high-dose penicillin, given both topically and systemically. *Chlamydia trachomatis* infection will be eradicated with chlortetracycline eye ointment and systemic erythromycin. Most other minor infections will respond to neomycin or chloramphenicol eye drops or ointment. When gonorrhea or chlamydia is diagnosed, both parents will require genital swabs and treatment.
Complications	Inadequate treatment of gonococcal ophthalmia may lead to corneal scarring and blindness. In developing countries, chlamydia frequently causes blindness from trachoma, but this is uncommon in developed countries. The reason for this different outcome from the same organism is unclear.

* drops → per vaginum delivery -only

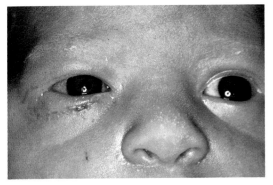

Fig. 127 Minor sticky eye with conjunctival inflammation.

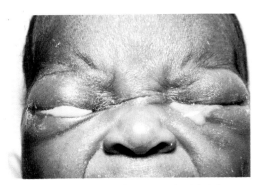

Fig. 128 Frank pus discharge in gonococcal ophthalmia.

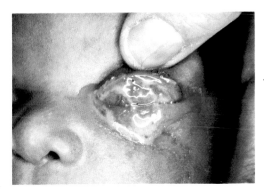

Fig. 129 Chlamydia ophthalmia.

Thrush

Synonyms

Monilia, candida.

Incidence

Superficial infection of the mouth or perineum is extremely common, particularly after antibiotic therapy.

Etiology

Fungal infection caused by *Candida albicans*.

Clinical features

Oral or perineal thrush is usually a trivial but distressing superficial infection. In the mouth, it appears as white plaques that cannot be wiped off without causing bleeding (Fig. 130). Sometimes, on visual inspection, it may be difficult to distinguish from milk immediately after a feed, but milk can always be easily wiped off. Perineal thrush gives a bright red confluent rash in the diaper area or around the anus. Typically, there are discrete ulcerated satellite lesions lying peripheral to the confluent rash (Fig. 131).

Management

Swabs or scrapings should be taken to confirm the diagnosis, although it is usually clinically obvious. Superficial thrush responds rapidly to topical nystatin or miconazole. Systemic candidiasis, although uncommon, may occur in ill preterm infants and responds poorly to antifungal agents.

Human immunodeficiency virus (HIV) infection

Incidence

Becoming more common as a result of the epidemic throughout the world. In Europe, intravenous drug-using mothers are most at risk. In Africa, the infection is largely transmitted heterosexually.

Clinical features

Most newborn babies with infection appear normal. Acquired immunodeficiency syndrome (AIDS) does not usually develop until the baby is several months old. At least 85% of the babies of HIV-positive mothers prove to be uninfected. It is necessary to wait about 18 months to be certain that the baby is antigen- and antibody-negative. Recurrent candida infection is a common early feature of AIDS.

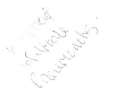

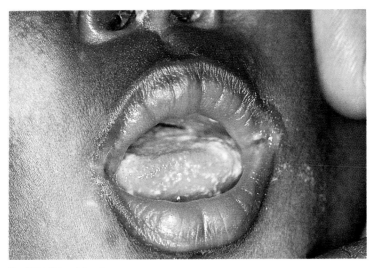

Fig. 130 Mild oral thrush.

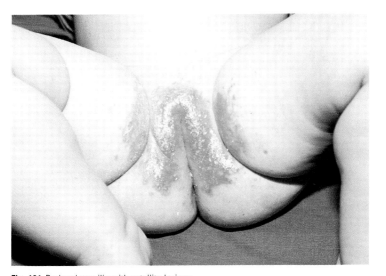

Fig. 131 Perineal monilia with satellite lesions.

Congenital rubella

Synonym	Rubella embryopathy.
Incidence	Depends on the state of immunity of the child-bearing population and the occurrence of rubella epidemics in the community.
Etiology	Rubella virus infection. Severe abnormalities occur with infection before 12 weeks' gestation.
Clinical features	Growth retardation with mental deficiency and microcephaly, deafness, cataracts, microphthalmia (Fig. 132), and congenital heart disease occur in severely affected infants. Hepatosplenomegaly, anemia, thrombocytopenic purpura (Fig. 133), and osteolytic lesions in long bones may be present.
Prevention	All young children are now immunized against rubella to reduce the frequency of rubella embryopathy in the future. Women without antibodies should be immunized when they are not pregnant.

Neonatal herpes infection

Incidence	Uncommon.
Etiology	*Herpes virus hominis*, usually type II virus, which is acquired by the infant during delivery through a genital tract with active herpes infection.
Clinical features	A generalized vesicular eruption (Fig. 134) occurs, and if encephalitis occurs, mortality is very high.
Prognosis	There is a high risk of neurologic abnormality and mental retardation among survivors.
Management	Systemic antiviral agents (acyclovir) may be helpful if commenced early in the disease.
Prevention	Elective cesarean section should be considered if active maternal genital herpes has been present in late pregnancy.

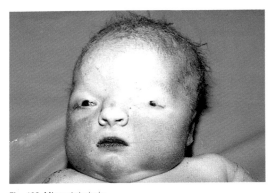

Fig. 132 Microphthalmia.

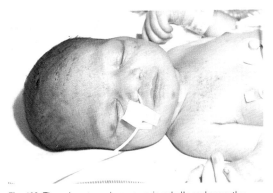

Fig. 133 Thrombocytopenic purpura in rubella embryopathy.

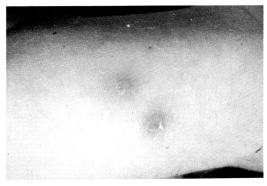

Fig. 134 Typical herpetic lesions.

Congenital chickenpox

Incidence

Chickenpox in pregnancy and in the newborn period is common. The fetus will be immune if the mother has had chickenpox. Serious neonatal illness is rare but occurs if the mother develops the rash of chickenpox within 48 h of delivery.

Clinical features

A newborn infant may develop the lesions of classic chickenpox just like the mother (Figs. 135 and 136). An infant may rarely have scars after infection in utero (Fig. 137).

Management

Hyperimmune zosterglobulin should be administered to the infant at birth if maternal chickenpox is likely. Babies who develop neonatal chickenpox should be given acyclovir to reduce the risk of complications, particularly pneumonitis.

Listeriosis

Incidence

The incidence of neonatal Listeriosis is reported as 13 cases/100,000 live births (roughly 30% of the total number of Listeria cases). The bacterium is present in many foods, such as soft unpasteurized cheeses or in salads.

Clinical features

The mother often has a mild febrile illness. The fetus may be infected in utero so that abortion or premature delivery is common. After birth, the baby often has a rash with discrete ulceration of the skin (Fig. 138). Pneumonia and meningitis are recognized features of the illness.

Management

Early diagnosis is essential so that appropriate antibiotic therapy can be used. Ampicillin is the drug of choice. With early treatment, intact survival should be possible.

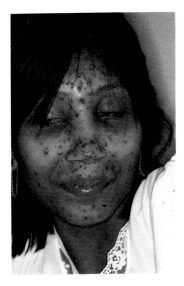

Fig. 135 Mother with chickenpox.

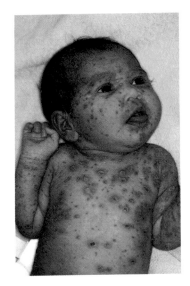

Fig. 136 Infant of mother in Figure 135, presenting with chickenpox.

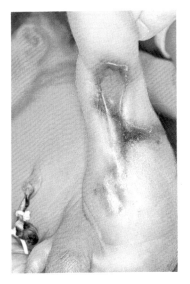

Fig. 137 Scars of intrauterine chickenpox.

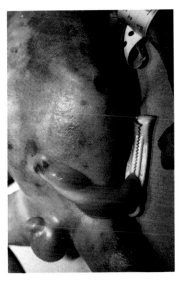

Fig. 138 Skin ulcers in listeriosis.

Cytomegalovirus (CMV)

Incidence

Incidence of congenital CMV is estimated at 0.5–2.0% of live births.

Clinical features

When the mother is infected, she usually has either a mild flu-like illness or no symptoms at all. Infected infants (Fig. 139) often have no abnormal features in the newborn period. They may be anemic, or have hepatosplenomegaly, purpura, jaundice, lymphadenopathy, intracranial calcification, and pneumonia. Microcephaly may be a feature. Deafness, mental handicap, cerebral palsy, and epilepsy may occur later.

Prognosis

Most infants with CMV infection have no sequelae. About 5% develop deafness, and 1% show more serious neurologic manifestations.

Toxoplasmosis

Incidence and transmission

Incidence of congenital Toxo plasmosis is estimated at 0.3–1.0 infant/1,000 live births. The infection is acquired from eating raw infected meat or from cat feces.

Clinical features

Infected infants may appear quite normal. Sometimes there is hepatosplenomegaly, purpura, jaundice, growth retardation, intracranial lesions and calcification (Fig. 140), chorioretinitis, and hydrocephalus. The neurologic damage may be very severe, although this is rare. Chorioretinitis seems to occur in all infected infants.

Diagnosis

Not all babies will be infected if a mother has an acute infection in pregnancy. Serologic evidence of infection can be obtained from the mother; blood samples from the baby will show whether toxoplasma-specific IgM is present. IgM-negative babies may still have an infection and may need to be followed for many months after birth to be certain that they are normal.

Management

Spiramycin is often used in pregnancy after proven infection and continued after birth. Pyrimethamine and sulfadiazine are used for infants but not in the immediate newborn period. Treatment is particularly important in chorioretinitis.

Prognosis

Variable. Many children only have eye lesions, but neurologic damage may be extremely severe, even though it is rare.

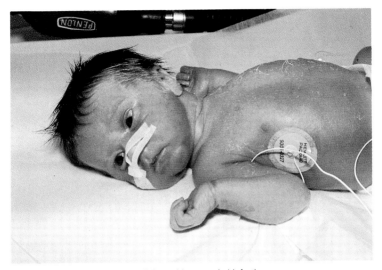

Fig. 139 Jaundice and purpura in infant with congenital infection.

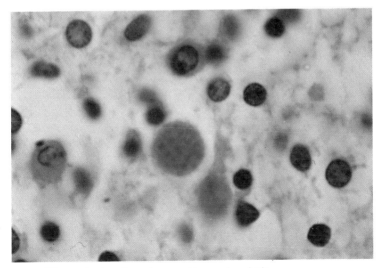

Fig. 140 Microscopic view of toxoplasma cyst in a newborn brain.

9 / Surgical problems

Umbilical hernia

Incidence

Common; 20% of all infants and 60% black infants. There is a higher incidence in preterm infants.

Clinical features

Central defect in the abdominal wall at the insertion of the umbilicus, with herniation of bowel into the redundant umbilical skin (Fig. 141). The hernia usually develops after the first week of life. On crying, straining, or coughing, the skin covering the bowel-filled hernia often becomes tense, shiny, and bluish. It is not painful but becomes more pronounced with crying. Umbilical hernias always reduce easily when the infant is lying quietly or when asleep.

Significance

Cosmetic deformity only. Strangulation is extremely rare in central umbilical hernias but may occur in paraumbilical hernias (defect in the linea alba separate from but adjacent to the umbilicus).

Management

Most close spontaneously within the first few years of life. Strapping does not hasten spontaneous resolution. Cosmetic surgery is occasionally required.

Umbilical granuloma

Incidence

Common.

Clinical features

A soft, spongy, and often pedunculated pink umbilical mass (Fig. 142), which is sometimes accompanied by a serosanguineous discharge.

Differential diagnosis

Careful inspection should exclude a persistent urachus or omphalomesenteric remnant.

Management

Application of silver nitrate to the granuloma or the pedunculated base until resolution occurs. Surgical excision is occasionally required.

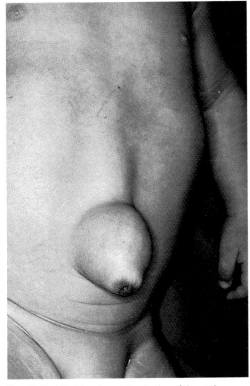

Fig. 141 Umbilical hernia and divarication of the recti.

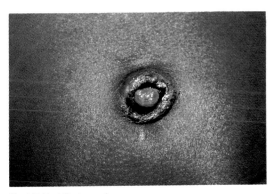

Fig. 142 Umbilical granuloma.

Inguinal hernia

Incidence

Indirect inguinal hernia is the most common condition requiring surgery during infancy: 1 in 50 live male births, with the greatest incidence in the first 3 months of life.

Etiology

Persistent patency of the processus vaginalis, accompanied by herniation of small bowel.

Clinical features

Intermittent swelling in the inguinal region or scrotum, often noticed after crying or straining (Fig. 143). Hernias are usually easily reducible, but when they become irreducible there is a high risk of strangulation.

Management

Surgical repair should be performed as soon as practicable after the diagnosis of an uncomplicated hernia because the risk of strangulation is high in young infants. Strangulation, with a tense, tender, and irreducible swelling sometimes accompanied by vomiting, abdominal distension, and signs of gut obstruction, is an indication for immediate surgery.

Hydrocele

Incidence

Common.

Etiology

Patency of the processus vaginalis.

Clinical features

A hydrocele is a painless, fluid-filled cyst anterior to the testis. The testis can usually be easily palpated within the scrotum. The hydrocele is brightly translucent (Fig. 144) and cannot be emptied by pressure, although it may vary in size. The swelling can be differentiated from a hernia because it does not extend up to the inguinal ring.

Management

Most hydroceles in infancy resolve spontaneously within the first year of life.

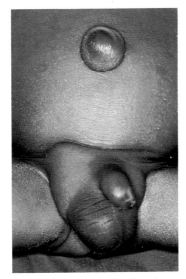

Fig. 143 Bilateral inguinal hernia and umbilical hernia.

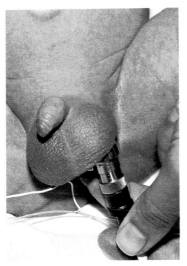

Fig. 144 Transillumination of hydrocele.

Hypospadias

Incidence

Glandular hypospadias is common (1 in 350 male infants).

Clinical features

The urethral orifice is situated on the ventral aspect of the penis at a site proximal to the normal opening (Fig. 145), with severity varying from a glandular orifice to a scrotal or perineal site. Hypospadias is usually accompanied by a redundant dorsal hooded prepuce (due to failure of fusion of the ventral foreskin) and is sometimes associated with ventral curvature called chordee (Fig. 146).

Management

Mild glandular hypospadias without chordee is usually insignificant, and surgery is not required unless there is meatal stenosis. Surgical repair is indicated if the orifice is situated proximal to the glans or if chordee is present: this can only be judged when the baby has an erection.

Circumcision should be delayed until corrective surgery is performed, as the prepuce may be required for urethroplasty.

Bladder exstrophy

Incidence

Very rare; more common in males.

Clinical features

Wide separation of the pubic symphysis with ventral herniation of the bladder, exposure of the bladder mucosa, and a deficiency of the pelvic floor leading to rectal prolapse (Fig. 147). The condition is often accompanied by epispadias, undescended testis, and an inguinal hernia. In the female, the clitoris is frequently septate or duplicated. Abnormalities of the kidneys are common.

Management

Surgical reconstruction is difficult. Continence is rarely achieved.

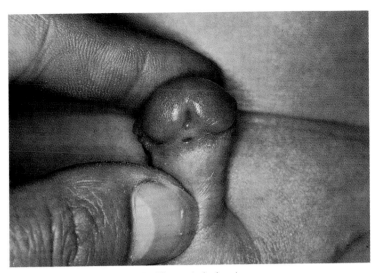

Fig. 145 Hypospadias with urethral orifice on shaft of penis.

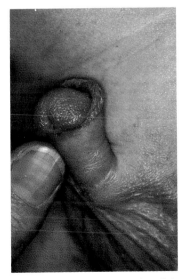

Fig. 146 Hypospadias with dorsal hooded prepuce.

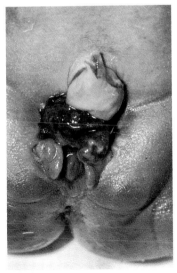

Fig. 147 Bladder exstrophy.

Necrotizing enterocolitis (NEC)

Incidence

Variable: more common in preterm infants. The condition has been found to be associated with birth asphyxia, umbilical catheterization, early feeding, and artificial milk formulas. Clusters of cases may occur.

Etiology

Unknown. The single most important risk factor is not ischemia but rather prematurity. Infants who develop NEC are thought to have an incompetent mucosal barrier, and an overgrowth of bacteria at the incompetent barrier leads to infection and progression of disease.

Pathology

Histologic evidence of impaired gut perfusion, bowel ischemia, and necrosis, usually affecting the terminal ileum, caecum, and proximal transverse colon.

Clinical features

Abdominal distension, vomiting, and the passage of bloody stools. NEC is sometimes accompanied by peritonitis, edema of the anterior abdominal wall, dilated abdominal veins, or a palpable mass (Fig. 148).

Invasion by gas-forming organisms or diffusion of intraluminal gas into the bowel wall gives rise to the pathognomonic sign of pneumatosis intestinalis (intramural bubbles of gas) on plain abdominal radiograph (Figs. 149 and 150). Portal venous gas (in addition to pneumatosis) is considered a pathognomonic finding of NEC on radiography. This can develop into a life-threatening situation in infants. They must be made NPO with a sump tube placed in the stomach to allow continuous suction for decompression. They must be cultured for any potential infection (blood, CSF, urine) and broad-spectrum antibiotics should be started. Often, these infants require vigorous volume resuscitation. They must have serial laboratory studies checked until their clinical status stabilizes. Serial radiographs watching for perforation are necessary until the baby is stable.

Course and prognosis

With conservative management, the mortality has improved, but gut obstruction secondary to adhesions or stricture may require surgical intervention at a later stage in approximately 25% of survivors.

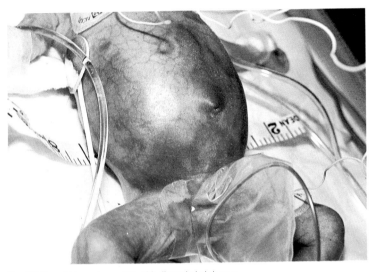

Fig. 148 Necrotizing enterocolitis with distended abdomen.

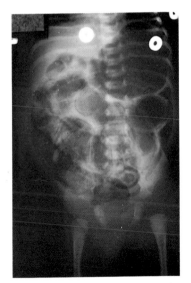

Fig. 149 Radiograph showing intramural gas.

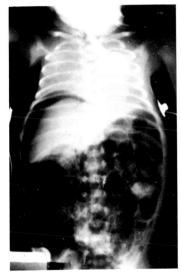

Fig. 150 Radiograph showing gas in the peritoneal cavity from perforation.

Exomphalos

Synonym Omphalocele.

Incidence Uncommon.

Etiology Unknown.

Pathology The defect arises as a fascial defect that develops as a result of a failure of the lateral, caudal and cranial abdominal embryonic folds to fuse appropriately. The bowel is nonrotated and fails to migrate back into the abdominal cavity. This defect involves the umbilical ring.

Clinical features This is a congenital herniation of abdominal viscera through midline abdominal wall defect with umbilical cord at apex and sometimes with a covering of peritoneum (Figs. 151 and 152). There is always a peritoneal sac over the bowel but it may be ruptured at time of delivery. Exomphalos can be differentiated from gastroschisis in which there is no sac and the umbilical cord and ring are not part of the defect; the cord always lies separately to the left of this defect.

Associations Other congenital abnormalities are common, particularly cardiac or bowel defects, and include cardiac, neurologic, skeletal, genitourinary and chromosomal (trisomy 13, trisomy 18) defects. There is also an association with Beckwith–Wiedemann syndrome. Bowel function is usually normal although there is a malrotation.

Management Surgical closure as soon as possible. The bowel should first be carefully inspected for stenosis or atresia, which often accompanies exomphalos. With large defects, definitive repair is often delayed until the peritoneal cavity is able to accommodate the contents. The sac and contents are usually enclosed in an artificial membrane, which is gradually reduced in size over a period of some weeks as the contents are slowly replaced into the abdominal cavity. There is a risk for increased fluid, protein, and heat loss from exposed viscera. Thermal regulation and careful fluid management are crucial.

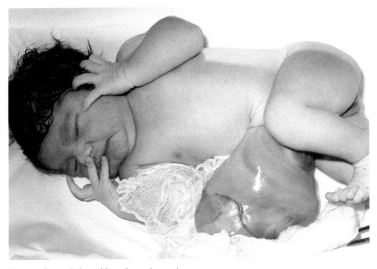

Fig. 151 Exomphalos with peritoneal covering.

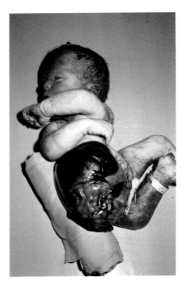

Fig. 152 Massive exomphalos with herniation of entire abdominal contents.

Imperforate anus

Synonyms Anal atresia, covered anus, rectal atresia.

Clinical features Imperforate anus (Figs. 153 and 154) is usually diagnosed during routine examination immediately after birth but occasionally presents later as intestinal obstruction or delayed passage of meconium.

Associations Other congenital abnormalities are found in approximately 60% of cases. Rectogenitourinary fistulas are common, particularly in high rectal atresia. Urinary tract infections are common, particularly when there is a fistula.

Management In the simplest cases, the covering of the anus can be incised. In the more usual cases, colostomy is performed in the neonatal period. A thorough search should be made for fistulas, particularly in females. Rectoplasty and a pull-through procedure are done later, at 6–12 months of age. Continence is achieved in approximately 70% of cases after final surgery.

Vaginal defects

Incidence Uncommon.

Clinical features Imperforate hymen is a rare condition that may present in the neonatal period with an accumulation of mucus beneath the imperforate membrane (mucocoplos) that bulges out between the labia minora. Paravaginal cysts (Fig. 155) may be confused with an imperforate hymen, but it is possible to pass a probe into the vagina alongside the cyst.

Management Imperforate hymen requires surgical drainage and excision of the membrane. Paravaginal cysts usually rupture spontaneously.

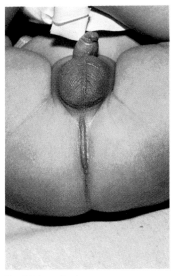

Fig. 153 Imperforate anus.

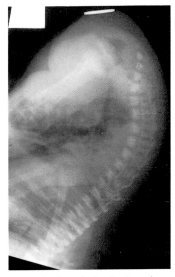

Fig. 154 Radiograph showing imperforate anus with high rectal atresia.

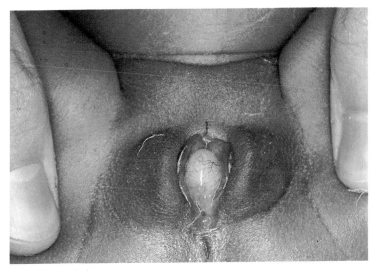

Fig. 155 Paravaginal cyst.

Diaphragmatic hernia

Occurs in 1 in 1,500 live births.

Failure of fusion or muscularization of the anterior and posterior leaves of the diaphragm. The condition is most commonly due to persistence of the pleuroperitoneal canal, usually on the left side and resulting in a posterolateral hernia through the foramen of Bochdalek.

Most cases are now recognized by ultrasound examination before birth.

Most diaphragmatic hernias are large and produce cardiorespiratory symptoms soon after birth. The signs and symptoms depend on the size of the hernia and include respiratory distress, cyanosis, dextrocardia, and scaphoid abdomen with reduced or absent abdominal contents (Fig. 156).

Pulmonary hypoplasia; gut anomalies.

Arrange for the mother's delivery in a perinatal center with a pediatric surgical service. Confirm the diagnosis with a chest radiograph after birth (Fig. 157). Preoperative decompression of the gut with a large nasogastric tube and mechanical ventilation may be required. Treat pulmonary hypertension. Delay the surgical repair of the diaphragmatic defect until the baby's condition is stable.

Mortality is high even after successful surgery. Survival depends on the severity of pulmonary hypoplasia. Better treatment of pulmonary hypertension and delayed surgery may improve survival.

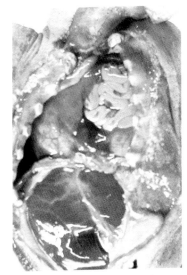

Fig. 156 Postmortem appearance of diaphragmatic hernia. (By courtesy of Dr. S. Gould.)

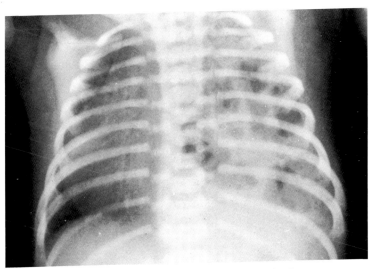

Fig. 157 Radiograph appearance of typical left-sided diaphragmatic hernia.

Preterm (1)

Definition

An immature infant of <37 weeks' gestation and birth weight usually <2,500 g. The very premature require intensive care (Fig. 158).

Incidence

In the U.S., 7.3% of live births are of low birth weight (<2,500 g). About two-thirds of these are preterm infants. Babies <1,500 g make up about 1% of births but nearly 50% of perinatal deaths.

Etiology

Often unknown. Sometimes, the infant has to be delivered early because of maternal complications of pregnancy such as pre-eclampsia or placenta previa. Preterm labor is often associated with cervical incompetence, multiple pregnancy, premature rupture of the membranes, or amnionitis.

Clinical features

It is possible to make an estimate of gestational age from a combination of external physical and neurologic signs. The preterm infant has poor muscle tone and tends to lie in a frog-like position. There is a relatively large head and prominent abdomen. Because the skull bones are soft and poorly mineralized, the head of the preterm infant often becomes narrow and elongated (Fig. 159), particularly if the infant is nursed with the head to one side. This deformity of the shape of the skull improves spontaneously in later infancy and is of no significance.

Skin creases are poorly developed, particularly on the soles of the feet (Fig. 160). Lanugo hair is often profuse in babies of 30–36 weeks' gestation but is less common in very preterm or more mature infants. It is usually most pronounced over the back and shoulders but may occur all over the body (Fig. 161). Ear cartilage is soft and deficient, and the pinna is poorly developed (Fig. 161), with little elastic recoil. ➡

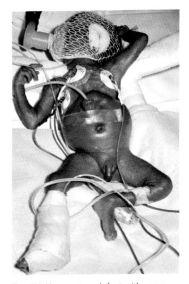

Fig. 158 Very preterm infant with some equipment of modern intensive care.

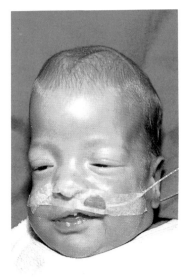

Fig. 159 Preterm infant with narrow, elongated head.

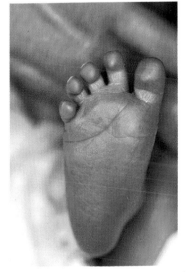

Fig. 160 Poorly developed skin creases on feet.

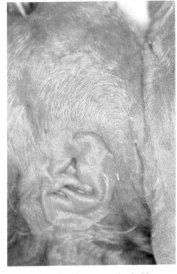

Fig. 161 Profuse lanugo and primitive ear development.

Preterm (2)

Clinical features (cont.)

The skin is often bright red, shiny, and transparent, with subcutaneous blood vessels readily visible (Fig. 162). The skin of the preterm infant is easily damaged by even minor trauma such as adhesive tape or transcutaneous electrodes. The nipple does not appear until 28 weeks' gestation, and breast tissue does not develop until after 34 weeks' gestation. The genitalia show major changes with advancing gestation. In female infants, the clitoris is relatively large with gaping of the vulva due to prominent labia minora (Fig. 163). In male infants, the scrotum is underdeveloped, and the testes may be undescended (Fig. 164).

Complications and associations

- Respiratory distress syndrome (hyaline membrane disease).
- Periventricular hemorrhage.
- Poor temperature control.
- Increased susceptibility to infection.
- Severe and prolonged physiologic jaundice.
- Feeding difficulties and inability to suck.
- Fluid and electrolyte imbalance.
- Retinopathy of prematurity.
- Chronic lung disease.

Course and prognosis

Mortality is still high in very preterm infants. Survival is uncommon under 24 weeks' gestation, but 60% of infants survive at 28 weeks and 95% at $\geq$30 weeks. With optimal care, >90% of preterm infants who survive the neonatal period have no serious neurologic handicap.

Periventricular leukomalacia with cysts alongside the ventricle is associated with a high incidence of neurologic disability.

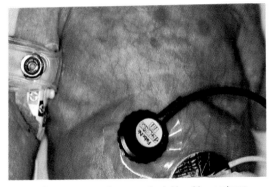

Fig. 162 Transparent, easily traumatized skin with prominent veins.

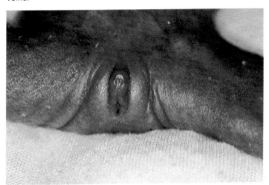

Fig. 163 Immature female genitalia with prominent labia minora and enlarged clitoris.

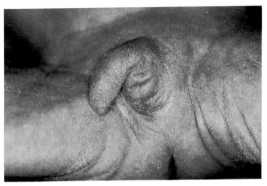

Fig. 164 Immature male genitalia with underdeveloped scrotum and undescended testis.

Small for gestational age (SGA)

Synonyms Small for dates; intrauterine growth retardation.

Definition Birth weight <10th centile for gestational age.

Incidence 2 in 100 live births are SGA and <2,500 g.

Etiology May be associated with placental insufficiency, maternal pre-eclampsia, hypertension or smoking, and intrauterine infection such as rubella.

Clinical features The most common SGA infants are usually long and thin, with dry peeling skin (Figs. 165 and 167) and long nails. Their physical appearance and behavior are appropriate for gestational age, not birth weight. Some SGA infants are uniformly small; they are at risk of perinatal asphyxia and often have meconium staining of the skin (Fig. 166), nails, and umbilical cord. Unless they are ill, SGA infants feed very well and require increased caloric intake. Their physiologic weight loss is usually insignificant, and they gain weight rapidly with adequate postnatal nutrition. They are at risk of hypoglycemia in the first few days after birth. Hypothermia may also occur.

Course and prognosis In the absence of intrauterine infection or neonatal hypoglycemia, SGA infants are usually of normal intelligence and development. Infants of low birth weight but appropriate head circumference and length for gestation usually achieve normal centiles for all aspects of growth later. If the head circumference, weight, and length are all low at birth, indicating long-standing intrauterine growth retardation, postnatal growth may always remain below the normal centiles.

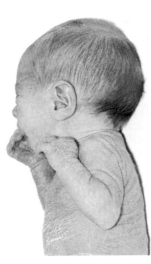

Fig. 165 Dry peeling skin of SGA infant.

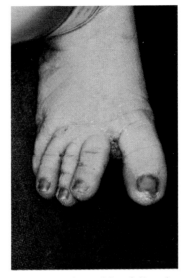

Fig. 166 Meconium staining of skin and nails.

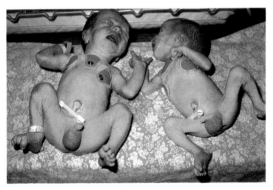

Fig. 167 SGA and normal twins.

Hyaline membrane disease (HMD) (1)

Synonym

Respiratory distress syndrome.

Incidence

The most common neonatal respiratory disease. Gestational age is the main determinant of HMD; at least 50% of infants <32 weeks' gestation develop the disease. About 70% of infants with a lecithin/sphingomyelin (L:S) ratio less than 1.5:1 develop HMD. It is extremely rare if the L:S ratio is greater than 2:1.

Etiology

Due to surfactant deficiency in the infant's lungs, HMD is more likely to develop in infants who suffer perinatal asphyxia and infants of diabetic mothers.

Clinical features

HMD presents with respiratory distress within 4 h of birth. The infant usually has tachypnea >60/min, an expiratory grunt, cyanosis, and sternal, intercostal, and subcostal recession (Fig. 168). After 4 h of age, HMD can usually be clearly distinguished from transient tachypnea due to delayed lung liquid resorption by a characteristic radiologic appearance. Chest X-ray shows a diffuse reticulogranular pattern due to atelectasis, and an air-bronchogram due to the air-filled major airways standing out as radiolucent areas (Fig. 169). In more serious HMD, the heart border may become obscured.

Course and prognosis

HMD gradually gets worse over the first 24–36 h as the infant tires and, if there are no complications, steadily improves from 48 h onward as surfactant is produced. Most infants with uncomplicated HMD recover by 7–10 days of age. ➡

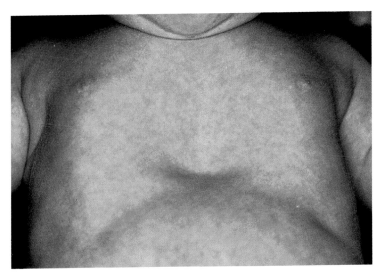

Fig. 168 Subcostal recession.

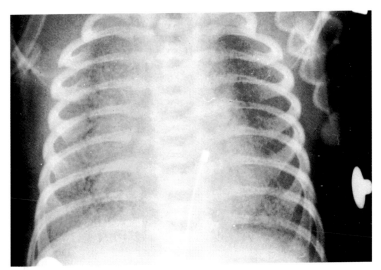

Fig. 169 Radiograph appearance of hyaline membrane disease.

Hyaline membrane disease (2)

Pneumothorax (Fig. 170) develops in up to 20% of infants with HMD, particularly if ventilation is required. In a small percentage of infants, pulmonary interstitial emphysema (Fig. 171), pneumomediastinum (Fig. 172), pneumopericardium, or bronchopulmonary dysplasia may develop. Such infants may need prolonged O_2 therapy; this is sometimes needed at home after discharge. Periventricular hemorrhage (PVH) is the major cause of death in preterm infants with HMD. The hemorrhage arises from the capillaries of the extremely vascular germinal layer of the floor of the lateral ventricle. Of infants <1,500 g, 40% suffer from PVH, which can be detected on ultrasound examination of the brain. Germinal layer hemorrhage or small PVH is of no serious significance. Hemorrhage that distends the ventricles, extends into brain substance, or causes posthemorrhagic hydrocephalus may be fatal or cause long-term neurologic sequelae.

The aim is to keep the infant alive and in good condition until natural surfactant synthesis occurs. Hypoxia, acidosis, and hypothermia will inhibit surfactant production. Exogenous surfactant, given into the trachea, is very effective. Oxygen and artificial ventilation are often necessary to maintain arterial PO_2 within the range 7–10 kPa (50–70 mmHg). Continuous monitoring of PaO_2 and frequent estimates of acid–base status are particularly important in the first few days when PVH often occurs.

Survival and long-term prognosis depend on gestation and the occurrence of complications. With improvement in ventilatory techniques in the past decade, PVH is now the main determinant of survival and neurologic handicap. With optimal care, <10% of preterm infants suffer major handicap.

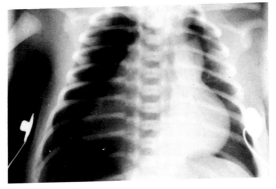

Fig. 170 Pneumothorax.

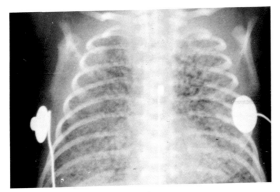

Fig. 171 Pulmonary interstitial emphysema.

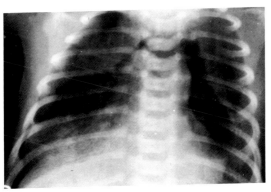

Fig. 172 Pneumomediastinum.

Nutrition

The major advantages of breast milk over formulas are its anti-infective properties and its better tolerance by infants. Fresh breast milk from the infant's own mother should be used whenever possible; pasteurization probably kills the white cells, and most anti-infective factors are destroyed by boiling. Breast-feeding (Fig. 173), or the use of expressed breast milk, is also psychologically important to the maternal–infant relationship. There are, however, physiologic limitations on nutrition in low-birth-weight infants. Particular difficulties may occur with low gastric volume tolerance, poor fat absorption, high energy requirement, and fluid and electrolyte imbalance in preterm infants.

Many infants are unable to suck because of immaturity or respiratory distress. They can be fed through an indwelling nasogastric tube, or by intermittent gavage feeding (Fig. 174), or a continuous infusion of milk may be delivered via a syringe pump. Continuous transpyloric feeding (Fig. 175) may be useful if apnea or vomiting occurs. Parenteral nutrition may be required in extremely small, immature, or very sick infants whose gut may not tolerate milk; it is best administered via a centrally placed Silastic catheter introduced through a peripheral vein. Low-birth-weight infants usually require high protein and water intake for normal weight gain. Additional supplements of sodium, iron, vitamins, calcium, phosphate-acid and folic acid are often necessary.

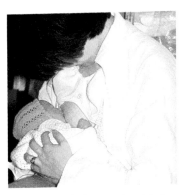

Fig. 173 Breast-feeding a preterm infant.

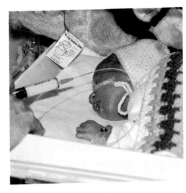

Fig. 174 Nasogastric feeding.

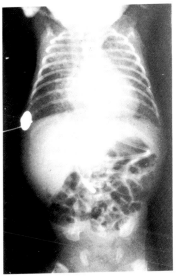

Fig. 175 Radiograph showing transpyloric tube for continuous milk infusion.

The family

Parental anxiety

Guilt and a sense of failure often accompany the birth of a low-birth-weight infant. The appearance, behavior, and illness of a preterm infant may be difficult for the parents to accept and understand. Discussion and explanation of the infant's condition and management, including the awesome equipment of the modern neonatal unit, will help to alleviate some of the uncertainty faced by the family—even though an accurate prediction of outcome cannot be made in the early stages.

Avoidance of separation

Unnecessary admission of well, low-birth-weight infants to a specialized neonatal unit should be avoided whenever possible, as such admission always results in separation for some members of the family. Open visiting for all family members, including siblings (Figs. 176 and 177), should be encouraged, and some contribution toward active participation in the infant's care is usually possible and is always satisfying. This may include nursing, cuddling, diaper changing, bathing (Fig. 178), and feeding all but the most ill preterm infant.

Even in the event of the death of the baby, parents are often best supported by allowing them to participate in the final decisions and moments of the infant's life.

Later problems

The high incidence of feeding and management problems is partly attributable to the immaturity of the infant and the fact that low-birth-weight infants are most often born to young mothers living in poor social conditions. With understanding and good support, many problems and parental anxieties can be overcome.

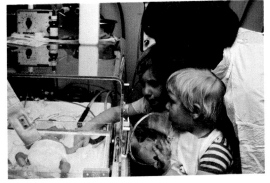

Fig. 176 Siblings visiting neonatal nursery.

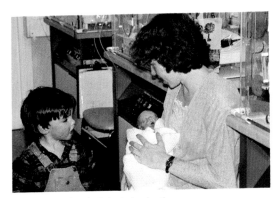

Fig. 177 Showing the baby to her brother.

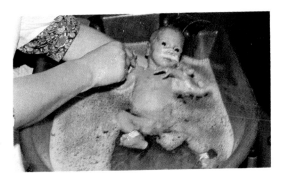

Fig. 178 Bathtime.

Index